Tai Chi Chuan Martial Applications

ADVANCED YANG STYLE

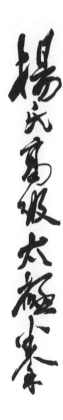

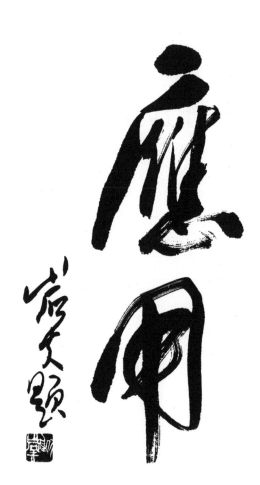

DR. YANG, JWING-MING

Tai Chi Chuan Martial Applications
ADVANCED YANG STYLE

YMAA Publication Center, Inc.
Wolfeboro, NH USA

YMAA Publication Center, Inc.
Main Office:
PO Box 480
Wolfeboro, New Hampshire, 03894
1-800-669-8892•info@ymaa .com • www.ymaa.com

ISBN: 9781594392993 (print) • ISBN: 9781594393044 (ebook)

3rd edition. Copyright © 1986, 1996, 2016 by Yang, Jwing-Ming
Copyedit by Leslie Takao and T. G. LaFredo
Caption Edit by Leslie Takao
Typesetting by Westchester Publishing Services
Cover design and drawings by Axie Breen
Photos by YMAA unless noted otherwise

20191114

Publisher's Cataloging in Publication

Names: Yang, Jwing-Ming, 1946-

Title: Tai chi chuan martial applications : advanced Yang style / Dr. Yang, Jwing-Ming. --

Description: 3rd ed. | Wolfeboro, NH USA : YMAA Publication Center, [2016] | Series: Tai chi chuan. | Revised edition of: Tai chi chuan martial applications: advanced Yang style tai chi chuan. 2nd ed., YMAA, c1996. | Some Chinese terms given in Chinese characters. | Includes bibliography and index. | Contents: Introduction -- Analysis of taijiquan techniques -- Taiji pushing hands -- Analysis of the taiji fighting set -- Taijiquan fighting strategy -- Conclusion -- Appendixes.

Identifiers: ISBN: 978-1-59439-299-3 (print) | 978-1-59439-304-4 (ebook) | LCCN: 2016950175

Subjects: LCSH: Tai chi. | Martial arts--Training. | Qi (Chinese philosophy) | Qi gong. | Martial arts--Health aspects. | Vital force. | Force and energy. | Martial arts--Psychological aspects. | BISAC: SPORTS & RECREATION / Martial Arts & Self-Defense. | BODY, MIND & SPIRIT / Healing / Energy (Qigong, Reiki, Polarity). | HEALTH & FITNESS / Exercise.

Classification: LCC: GV504 .Y363 2016 | DDC: 796.815/5--dc23

Editorial Notes

Romanization of Chinese Words

The interior of this book primarily uses the Pinyin romanization system of Chinese to English. In some instances, a more popular word may be used as an aid for reader convenience, such as "tai chi" in place of the Pinyin spelling, taiji. Pinyin is standard in the People's Republic of China and in several world organizations, including the United Nations. Pinyin, which was introduced in China in the 1950s, replaces the older Wade-Giles and Yale systems.

Some common conversions are found in the following:

Pinyin	Also spelled as	Pronunciation
qi	chi	chē
qigong	chi kung	chē gōng
qin na	chin na	chǐn nǎ
gongfu	kung fu	gōng foo
taijiquan	tai chi chuan	tī jē chǔén

For more information, please refer to *The People's Republic of China: Administrative Atlas, The Reform of the Chinese Written Language,* or a contemporary manual of style.

Formats and Treatment of Chinese Words

Transliterations are provided frequently: for example, *Five Animal Sport (Wu Qin Xi,* 五禽戲). In some cases, transliterated Chinese terms have the same spelling as English words. When this causes ambiguity, the editors place the Chinese terms in italics.

Chinese persons' names are presented mostly in their more popular English spelling. Capitalization is according to the *Chicago Manual of Style,* 16th edition. The author or publisher may use a specific spelling or capitalization in respect to the living or deceased person. For example, Cheng, Man-ch'ing can be written as Zheng Manqing.

Photographs

Many photographs include motion arrows to help show the starting position of the body motion.

Contents

Foreword By Grandmaster Liang, Tung-Tsai

Even though Dr. Yang, Jwing-Ming (楊俊敏) is still a young man, he has accomplished a great deal. He has earned a Ph.D. degree and has intensively studied and mastered the martial arts, both the hard and soft styles, along with forming the Yang's Martial Arts Association (YMAA) and compiling many valuable books.

Dr. Yang surely follows in the footsteps of the Yang style founder, Yang Lu-Chan (楊露禪), who also first studied the Shaolin hard styles and then later studied and mastered the soft style of T'ai Chi Ch'uan. Dr. Yang stimulates this tradition, which will surely bear the fruit of high achievement within the martial arts for him. Although Dr. Yang and myself have not personally met before, we both share a common affinity, that is, we both learned the Shaolin Chin Na from the same teacher, Master Han, Ching-Tang (韓慶堂).

After receiving this second Volume of *Advanced Yang Style Tai Chi Chuan: Martial Applications* (New Title: *Tai Chi Chuan Martial Applications*), I am indeed impressed. Both volumes one and two lay a solid foundation for the internal and self-defense applications of T'ai Chi Ch'uan. Everybody should read his books. So I am honored that I am writing this foreword to his new book. My two favorite students, Stuart Alve Olson and Jonathan Russell, both of whom have a friendship with Dr. Yang, originally presented me with the idea of writing a few words of introduction to this book. It is also my understanding that Jonathan Russell was instrumental in helping Dr. Yang become established in Boston shortly after I left that city to semi-retirement. So now it is my turn to help establish his book. It is my sincere hope that everybody learns something from Dr. Yang, Jwing-Ming in order to get some benefit from his intensive study and practice of the martial arts. He is a youth of great promise! By constantly studying and practicing the martial arts, in the near future Dr. Yang will reach the highest level, and then at once his name will be well known all over the world. Now let us rub our eyes and see!

Tung-Tsai Liang (梁棟材)
May, 1986

Preface (First Edition, 1986)

In Volume 1 of *Advanced Yang Style Tai Chi Chuan* (re-titled: *Tai Chi Chuan Martial Power*, 3rd Edition) we discussed the most important part of taijiquan: the principles and theory. We also translated and discussed the ancient Chinese poetry and songs that contain the accumulated experience and understanding of dozens of generations of taijiquan masters. The taijiquan beginner usually finds it very difficult to understand the deeper meaning of these writings, but as you accumulate experience you will gradually begin to grasp these keys. Therefore, you should continue to study and ponder, and one day you will understand the real value of these written secrets.

A major part of the theory of taijiquan's martial applications is involved with the use of jing (勁). Hopefully *Tai Chi Chuan Martial Power* has given you a good understanding of this subject. The theory of jing and its training methods have been kept secret for centuries. *Tai Chi Chuan Martial Power* is the first extensive discussion of this subject in English. I sincerely hope it will open the door to the research and study of jing, and make the general public aware of this neglected aspect of taijiquan.

If you understand the principles and theory of taijiquan and its jing, but do not know the martial techniques, your martial art is still half empty. It is as if you had learned how a car works, but not how to drive it. It cannot be denied that understanding the theory will help you to progress faster. However, since every form in the sequence was carefully designed to most efficiently attack and defend, you will also profit greatly from researching the application of each form to discover its potential and why it was designed just so. Once you have learned the martial applications, you still are not ready to use then in a real fight. You are in the position of someone who knows how to drive a car, but does not yet have any actual experience. In order to make the techniques usable, you must constantly practice them with a partner. Pushing hands and the fighting set were designed to resemble a real fight, and they give you the opportunity to apply the principles and theories you have learned. It is through this kind of mutual interaction of theory and practice that you become a taijiquan martial artist.

In this book, applications for every taijiquan form will be discussed in Chapter 2. This will lay the foundation of your knowledge of the martial aspect of taijiquan. Chapter 3 discusses the theory and training of pushing hands, and presents some of the martial applications that can be drawn from the movements of this exercise. Taiji ball training, which is commonly used to train certain jing, is also included in this chapter. Once you have obtained the fundamental keys of pushing hands, you will want to practice the taijiquan fighting set in Chapter 4. This set resembles real fighting, and it teaches you to set up your strategies as well as gives you further experience in the applications.

Finally, Chapter 5 will discuss the general rules and methods of fighting strategy, which will help you to further improve yourself through your own practice and research.

Dr. Yang, Jwing-Ming
1986

Preface (Second Edition, 1996)

After this book was first published in 1986, it significantly stimulated Western taijiquan society. From this book and the book *Tai Chi Chuan Martial Power 3rd Edition* (formerly titled *Advanced Yang Style Tai Chi Chuan, Volume One*), taijiquan practitioners in the West began to reevaluate the meaning and the value of taijiquan. Not only that, countless taijiquan practitioners began to search for the root and the essence of every movement in the form.

If we trace the origins of taijiquan, we see that it was created for self-defense. The health benefits were only a side effect of this art. But because of taijiquan's efficiency in maintaining health, it became one of the most popular meditative relaxation exercises both in the East and the West. Unfortunately, the martial applications of taijiquan were ignored in favor of the health aspects.

The result of this ignorance was the loss of the essence and the root of the original taijiquan. Only by understanding the martial applications can the meaning of every movement be felt profoundly, and the spirit of each posture be manifested correctly. Many readers have expressed that through reading this book, they now understand the crucial concepts and theories of the martial applications. From this understanding, they can apply what they have learned to the styles they practice.

You should understand that it does not matter which style of Chinese martial arts you have learned. If you trace the original root of the art, the basic fighting principles and theory remains the same. The Dao of self-defense is only one. According to a Chinese saying: "The Dao is the one which threads through (i.e., mutual co-related)" (道一以貫之). This implies that the universal rule of the Dao is the only rule. If you understand this Dao, you can apply it to everything in this universe.

Naturally, this Dao is understood as the theory and principle of yin (陰) and yang (陽). If you understand yin and yang thoroughly, you can apply it to anything in nature.

However, where does yin and yang originate? If we look at the *Yi Jing* (*The Book of Changes*, 易經), it is said: "What is taiji (i.e., grand ultimate)? It is originated from wuji (i.e., no extremity) and is the mother of yin and yang." From this you can see that taiji is between wuji and yin and yang (two poles). Taiji is the force that makes wuji divide into yin and yang. When we apply this idea into taijiquan, thinking becomes the motive force dividing the wuji into yin and yang. Therefore, without the mind or thinking, the movements in taijiquan have no meaning. And because taijiquan was conceived as a martial art, we see that this thinking or mind is the mind of defense; in other words, a sense of enemy.

In order to make every movement of taijiquan meaningful, you must first know the martial applications. Only then can your thinking be clear and the spirit of the form be manifested accurately. Therefore, if you are serious in searching out the root and the essence of taijiquan, you must study the martial applications. Only then can higher-level understanding be obtained.

In this new edition there are a few revisions:

1. In order to match the Romanization system currently used in China, all of the Chinese words in English follow the Pinyin system.
2. A glossary has been added.
3. Chinese words are included whenever it is necessary.

Since this book was first published, I have written twelve more books about qigong and Chinese martial arts. Among them, a few titles are highly recommended to those readers who are interested in learning more about Chinese taijiquan and qigong. These titles are:

1. *The Root of Chinese Chi Kung.* A clear, in-depth study of Chinese qigong practice. From this book, you can develop a clear understanding of your taijiquan and qigong practice.
2. *The Essence of Tai Chi Chi Kung.* This book was written to help interested taijiquan practitioners understand the inner side of taijiquan practice. From this book, you will be able to grasp the essence of taiji qigong practice.
3. *Taiji Chin Na.* Never before revealed to Western society, the grabbing and seizing techniques (i.e., chin na) of taijiquan are presented. This book is for those taijiquan practitioners who want to know more about the martial applications of taijiquan.
4. *The Essence of Shaolin White Crane.* Though the title of this book does not appear to be related to *taijiquan*, in fact, this book contains the most complete theory of Chinese martial qigong training—from the hard styles to the very soft styles, such as taijiquan. This book is highly recommended.

I hope this new edition brings you a better understanding of the essence of taijiquan. In order to promote this art to its highest level, we need all talented and experienced taijiquan masters to open their minds and share their knowledge through publications and instruction. Only then will this profound art continue to grow, and be assured of a bright future.

Dr. Yang, Jwing-Ming
1996

Preface (Third Edition, 2016)

Since this book was first published in 1986, taijiquan development has truly entered a new era. In the 1980s, most practitioners were only interested in health and consequently trained taijiquan only for relaxation. However, another group of practitioners has since emerged, and they have been hungrily searching for the hidden meanings and essence behind every taijiquan movement. They realized that without this knowledge and understanding, taijiquan is reduced to nothing more than a dance, a light exercise for relaxation, or a mere display of aesthetics. Although taijiquan health practitioners still trump traditionalists in numbers, those searching for the deeper root of the art have been steadily growing, especially in the last twenty years.

Taijiquan means the "fist of taiji." The "taiji" in taijiquan is actually the mind, and quan, or "fist," refers to the martial arts aspect of the practice. Therefore, taijiquan actually means the "fist of the mind." This is a crucial key to understanding taijiquan practice as a whole. Only when the mind is relaxed can your body be relaxed, and only when the body is relaxed can a practitioner truly realize the full potential of the entire art. In martial arts society, the final stage of martial arts training is almost always of the mind. This is because the mind is arguably the most difficult thing to master. One aspect that must be trained is developing a realistic and practical sense of opponent. The mind must be able to naturally sense an opponent and react appropriately with the right timing. All taijiquan movements were created for either offense or defense, so sense of opponent is of the utmost importance in taijiquan training. Sense of opponent raises spirit, focuses the mind, and allows qi to be led strongly throughout the body for efficient and powerful physical manifestations. You can see that without knowing the martial root of taijiquan (i.e., martial applications), the practice of taijiquan will be shallow.

Since the first edition of this book was published in 1986, countless taijiquan practitioners have contacted me to express their appreciation to me for writing this book and making it available to the general public. This motivated me to diligently continue my research and practice, eventually leading me to write and publish more than three dozen books and several instructional videos. I have been a martial arts author and teacher for more than forty years now. These publications constitute my lifetime of practice thus far. I highly recommend those who are interested in knowing more about taijiquan and qigong to take a look at my past works. Although I am only able to publish a small fraction of the knowledge out there based on my experience, I have seen many people reach what I consider to be a deep level of understanding simply through a very disciplined regime of practice and reading. I hope to offer everything that I can through my teachings, and I hope they will help you find your path in your training.

For this edition, I have double-checked that the concepts written in 1986 are still accurate according to my understanding and experience over the past three decades. In addition, I have added more Chinese characters in the text because the Chinese language has become so popular in this new century.

Dr. Yang, Jwing-Ming
YMAA California Retreat Center
May 18, 2015

Chapter 1: Introduction

1-1. General Introduction

The best way of studying a profound scientific subject is through both theory and experiment. Theory is the foundation of the entire study, and it is the theory that generates the principles and rules. These, in turn, lead to the creation of a prototype model for experimentation, which shows whether the theory and principles were accurate as originally stated. After many experiments and experiences, you can then confirm the accuracy of the theory and, if necessary, go back to modify the theory and principles. Again, you construct experiments based on the new modified theory and principles. It might take you many repeated cycles of theoretical research and experimental study before you can finally state your conclusions.

The same principle applies to taijiquan (太極拳). Taiji (太極) is based on the profound Daoist philosophies of yin (陰)/yang (陽), and the bagua (八卦), and it has been refined over more than one thousand years of research, study, and experimentation by many thousands of taijiquan martial artists. Even though a great deal has been passed down through the generations by teaching and writing, many taijiquan masters still feel that they have not learned the complete art. The more they dig, the deeper they feel the theory is. What is sad to see today is that the available knowledge is gradually dying out. Most taijiquan practitioners are more interested in the health aspect of taijiquan, rather than the martial side.

Taijiquan was originally created for martial purposes, and every form has its special martial applications. Many different styles have been created over the years, and although they are based on the same fundamental theory and principles, every style has its own characteristic specialties and applications. For example, a taijiquan style that has large postures might have different techniques and strategy than a style with small postures. However, regardless of the different emphasis, principles such as using the soft against the hard never change.

Learning the martial applications in the taijiquan sequence is just like learning the functions of the equipment in a car. After you have learned the function of everything in the car, you then take it for a drive and try everything out. The same principle is followed in taijiquan. After you have learned the techniques, you must experiment with them.

The taijiquan solo sequence is the foundation of all the martial techniques. Each movement or posture was carefully designed with the most appropriate stance for the intended strategic action, whether defensive or offensive. If you understand the applications and practice conscientiously, you will gain the necessary qi (氣) flow, jing (勁) expression, mental calmness, and—most important of all—sense of enemy. Once you understand taijiquan theory and principles and have mastered these techniques, you will need a partner for practice and experimentation. Pushing hands is the first step in making the applications alive and practical, and also introduces some applications that are not included in the solo sequence. After you have practiced pushing hands for some time, you should start training in a way that is more similar to a real fight. The two-person fighting set was designed for this purpose. It helps you learn how to analyze the situation, strategy, movements, and techniques of a real fight. Finally, you should start free-fighting training.

In this book, the author will discuss only the typical martial applications of the Yang style with large forms and low postures. There are more than 250 techniques in the 37 postures. This means that each posture has an average of six to seven techniques. Chapter 2 will discuss some of the typical applications of each technique known to the author. The deeper and more complicated applications will be omitted due to lack of space, and more importantly the difficulty of conveying the subtleties of the movements with the written word. However, if you study seriously and research carefully, you should be able to use your knowledge of the more basic techniques to discover the deeper levels of application. If the style you have learned is different from the style in this book, you can still use this book to gain ideas to adapt to your own style.

Chapter 3 will introduce the training for the heng (哼) and ha (哈) sounds, and the fundamentals of taiji ball training, which many taijiquan practitioners use to train their sensing and sticking capability. Last, taiji pushing hands will be reviewed. After you have mastered pushing hands, you should go on to the two-person fighting set in chapter 4. The various possible applications will be analyzed. Finally, chapter 5 will summarize the fighting strategy of taijiquan.

Even when you have mastered the techniques in this book, you are still not at the end of your study. In fact, you are only at the beginning of your research into martial applications. How much you learn and how far you progress is up to you. This book offers you the key to the treasure, but it cannot give you the treasure itself. You have to open the gate and step in, and search for the treasure by yourself. You might fail because of discouragement, impatience, or lack of perseverance. You might fall, only to stand up and continue. You might get injured from the thorns on the path. But you must understand that every time you fall, every time you get hurt from the thorns, it is always exactly what you need to gain experience. The more you experiment and the more experience you accumulate, the deeper your understanding of the theory will be. The more you carefully ponder, the clearer your understanding will be.

1-2. Becoming a Proficient Taijiquan Martial Artist

Once you have mastered the basic theory and fundamental techniques, you have reached a level where you are qualified to share and discuss your knowledge with others. You should be capable of teaching someone without too much deviation from the right path. The best way to start your teaching career is to be an assistant instructor for an experienced master for several years. Under his supervision, you will learn how to teach, but most important of all, you will be able to access his experience and pick up the many small points that do so much to fill out your knowledge. After a few years, you should start teaching on your own. Teaching is the best way to learn and become a proficient taijiquan martial artist. Through teaching, you learn how to analyze, how to explain, and how to set up a training schedule. After a few years of doing this, you will be able to create something of value and add to the store of taijiquan knowledge.

It is the urge to teach that has been responsible for taijiquan's being passed down from generation to generation. A master earns respect from sharing his knowledge with his students. Through his teaching and research, he also gains the friendship of those who share his interest and enthusiasm.

If you are hoping and planning to become a taijiquan master, there are several points that you should always remember:

1. Know the History

History is experience. If you do not know the past, you will be lost in the future. The past gives spiritual stimulation. From the past, you know your source and root. Knowing the history of taijiquan is the obligation of every practitioner who is willing to carry the responsibility of continuing the long tradition of the art.

A desire to know the history of the art indicates enthusiasm and a depth of interest in the art that will lead to profound knowledge. Remember, history is like a mirror that helps you to see yourself. It shows you the right way to the future.

2. Know the Theory and Principles

Every martial style is based on its own theory and principles. Taijiquan has its own unique principles, and if you disobey them, you are no longer doing taijiquan. Fortunately, these theories and principles have been passed down for generations through oral instruction or written documents. In order to be qualified as a taijiquan instructor, you must study all these documents and understand them. They are presented in the book *Tai Chi Chuan Martial Power*, from YMAA Publication Center, along with commentary.

3. Know What You Are Doing

Once you know the history and principles, you should ask yourself a few questions such as the following: Have I practiced these martial applications long enough so that

I can use them naturally whenever necessary? Do I have a good training schedule for my students and myself? How well do I know what I am doing? All in all, am I qualified to be a taijiquan master?

If your answers to these questions are negative, your teaching may earn you more shame than honor. When your qualifications are limited, you must work to improve yourself and your teaching. Be humble, and keep researching and pondering. Practice and discuss with your taijiquan friends, participate in seminars and workshops, and most important of all, make friends with all taijiquan stylists. Never be afraid to be humble and ask for other people's ideas and experiences. When you practice, keep digging and plowing, and never be satisfied with what you have already done. Look forward and not behind, and one day, you will harvest more than others. Then you will become a master.

4. Know What Other Instructors Are Doing

In order to become a real master, you need to know not only yourself, but also others. When you understand other styles, you can understand your own style better and evaluate it more objectively. You can evaluate how good it is and where its limitations are. Every style has its own specialties, so if you think some style is not as good as yours, it might just be that your knowledge of that style is still shallow. Also, when you see a style that seems better than yours, don't give up your style for it. That would be throwing away all the time and effort you have spent on it. After all, once you have invested a lot of time in this new style, you may find that there is nothing beneath the surface glitter that initially attracted you. If you believe that your style and your personal level of ability are superior to others, you must beware of losing your humility, for this may cause you to lose your enthusiasm for learning.

Sometimes you may hear of a martial artist who has studied only ten years but claims to have mastered five or even ten styles. Because it usually takes at least ten years of daily practice to master one style, such a person has probably studied each style only very superficially. Consider carefully whether you want to really master one or two styles, or whether you prefer learning a limited portion of ten or more styles. It is best to pick a style you believe is best for you, and to dig in and really learn it. If you learn one style to its fullest, you will be able to understand other styles more deeply and will be able to add substantial elements from other styles.

5. Know Your Students

Knowing your students is almost as important as knowing yourself. The questions you must ask about each student are as follows: What is his motivation in learning taijiquan? Can I trust this student? Is this student patient and persevering enough to fulfill his goals? If I teach him, will I be wasting my time? When this student has finished learning from me, will he continue his study from other sources? Will he become a good master in the future? Does he have good morality?

You must ask yourself these questions before you invest time and energy in any student. A student must first show interest, enthusiasm, respect, and loyalty. Then he must demonstrate strong will, patience, and perseverance to carry on the training. In other words, a student must show that he is worthy of your trust and teaching. In Chinese martial society, there is a saying: "A student will look for a good master for three years, and a master will test a student for three years." It is also said: "A master would prefer to spend ten years finding a good and trustworthy student instead of spending three years teaching ten untrustworthy students." When you teach a good student, he will pass down the art correctly. You can share your knowledge without hesitation, and can research and discuss with him without worrying that you may be betrayed. Sometimes a student, once he has finished learning from a master, starts to criticize or even scoff at his master in public. He does not realize that he is betraying his own root and foundation. Therefore, when you choose a student, you must be very cautious. A moral student will teach honestly, correctly, and loyally. He will pass down the traditional art correctly, but he will also add his own creative ideas. An immoral student will just hurt society and downgrade the martial art.

1-3. How to Use This Book

As mentioned before, this book explains only the martial applications of the Yang style using large forms and low postures, and so they are not necessarily directly applicable to the taijiquan style you have learned. Despite that, this book can still offer you a number of benefits. First, this book can give you the inspiration to investigate the applications in your style. Second, because the basic defense principles and theories are the same in every style, you may learn to analyze the forms in your own system and discover the applications. This book may also offer some insights into the higher levels of your style. Third, once you understand the martial applications in the Yang style, the similarities and differences may help you to better understand your own style.

In order to learn the trick of the martial applications of taijiquan, you must know how to analyze the postures. Once you have learned this, you can then apply the same basic principles and theories to any style. This is what is known as learning how to change a rock into a piece of gold instead of just taking the gold, and it is what separates a master from the average martial artist.

When you analyze a technique, you should keep the following in mind:

1. Perceive what.
2. Know how.
3. Understand why.
4. Predict when.

To really master the art, you should observe the following:

1. Discuss with your partners and ponder.
2. Practice from slow to fast.
3. Seek the applications in your own style.
4. Continue to research and ponder for the rest of your life.
5. Experiment with the techniques you have studied and analyzed.

Chapter 2: Analysis of Taijiquan Techniques

2-1. Introduction

Before we analyze the Yang-style taijiquan sequence, we would first like you to understand how martial sequences are created and what purposes they serve. Sometimes people who lack this understanding tend to view the taijiquan sequence as a dance or abstract movement. A proper understanding of the root of the art will help you practice in the most effective way.

A martial sequence is a combination of many techniques, constructed in the imagination of the creator to resemble a real fight. The creator of a sequence must be an expert in the style and experienced enough to see the advantages and disadvantages of a form, technique, or even just a step or stance. Within a martial sequence are hidden the secret techniques of a specific style. Chinese martial sequences contain two or three levels of fighting techniques. The first level is the obvious applications of the movements, and contains the fundamentals of the style.

The second level is deeper and is usually not obvious in the movements of a sequence. For example, a form might contain a false stance at a particular spot. This stance allows the practitioner to kick when necessary, but this kick may not actually be done in the sequence. Experienced martial artists can usually see through to this second level of applications.

The third level is the hardest to see, but it usually contains the most effective techniques of the style. These third-level techniques often require more movement or steps than are actually shown in the sequence, and must be explained and analyzed by the master himself. Therefore, a Chinese martial sequence has several purposes:

1. A sequence is used to preserve the essence of a style and its techniques. It is just like a textbook that is the foundation of your knowledge of a style.

2. A sequence is used to train a practitioner in the particular techniques of a style. When a student regularly practices a sequence, he can master the techniques and build a good foundation in his style.

3. A sequence is used to train a student's patience, endurance, and strength, as well as stances, movements, and jing (勁) (i.e., martial power).

4. A sequence is also used to help the student build a sense of enemy. From routinely practicing with an imaginary opponent, you can make the techniques alive and effective in a real fight.

The taijiquan sequence was created for these same purposes. However, as an internal style, it also trains the coordination of breath with qi, and qi with movement. For this reason, taijiquan training is slow in the beginning and then gradually incorporates speed.

Even though Yang-style taijiquan has many different versions that can have 24, 37, 81, 88, 105, or more postures (depending, in part, upon the method of counting), it actually contains only 37 to 40 fundamental martial techniques. These fundamental techniques form the basis of more than 250 martial applications. Within the sequence, many postures or fundamental techniques are repeated one or more times. There are several reasons for this:

1. To increase the number of times you practice the techniques that are considered more important and useful. This, naturally, will help you learn and master them more quickly. For example, wardoff (peng, 掤), rollback (lu, 攦), press (ji, 擠), and push (an, 按), which are considered the most basic fighting forms, are repeated eight times in the long sequence.

2. To increase the duration of practice for each sequence. When early taijiquan practitioners found that the original short sequence was not long enough to satisfy their exercise and practice needs, they naturally increased the time of practice by repeating some of the forms. Doing this lengthened sequence once in the morning and/ or evening is usually sufficient for health purposes. However, if you also intend to practice taijiquan for martial purposes, you should perform the sequence continuously three times, both morning and evening if possible. The first time is for warming up, the second is for qi transportation training, and the third time is for relaxed recovery.

As mentioned before, there are more than 250 martial techniques within the taijiquan sequence. These techniques are divided into three main categories: downing the enemy (i.e., wrestling) (shuai, 摔), joint locking (qin na or chin na, 擒拿), and cavity strike (ti, da, 踢、打). In fact, almost all Chinese martial art styles train these three categories, but taijiquan remains unique in that it specializes in doing them with relaxed muscles. This relaxation increases your sensitivity to the opponent's movement and intentions, which allows you to use the soft against the hard and to conquer strength with weakness. Because of its qi support and soft jing training, muscular strength becomes unimportant. It is for this reason that taijiquan's martial applications are much harder to understand and train. A qualified master is almost a necessity to lead the student to an understanding of the techniques and of the coordination of jing and qi with the techniques.

It is impossible to keep all the techniques in your conscious mind. In order to learn these techniques well enough to use them correctly and automatically, you must learn how to analyze and dissect them. You must learn how to figure out why a technique is done a particular way, and you must learn how to evaluate your options when your opponent makes a particular move. For example, when your opponent raises his arm to block, you should be familiar with the various techniques available to you, and you must understand why you should do this particular technique and not that one.

If you continue your analysis under a good instructor, you will be able to grasp the key to taijiquan martial applications, and will then find it unnecessary to memorize all the techniques. This is what is called "Learning the trick of changing a rock into a piece of gold, instead of just taking the gold." The first way is alive and unlimited; the latter is dead and limited. Once you have learned the trick of analysis from your instructor, you will then be able to continue to develop and learn on your own.

In this chapter, the thirty-seven fundamental taijiquan techniques will be analyzed and discussed. It is impossible to list all the possible applications of each technique. The examples, which include techniques from all three levels, are meant only to guide the interested taijiquan martial artist to the gate. To pass beyond this point and enter the temple requires that you continue to study and research on your own.

The next section of this chapter will discuss the principles of taijiquan martial application. This section will help you lay the foundation of knowledge for the martial techniques. The last section will analyze and discuss possible applications for each taijiquan form in the sequence.

2-2. General Principles of Taijiquan Techniques

In Chinese martial arts, the fighting techniques can usually be classified into three categories: downing the enemy (shuai jiao, 摔跤) (i.e., Chinese wrestling), joint locking (qin na or chin na, 擒拿), and cavity strike (dian xue, 點穴) (i.e., kicking and punching to cavities, ti and da, 踢、打). Many techniques are a combination of two of these categories. Very often, one category will be used immediately after another. For example, qin na control is very often used together with downing the enemy to make the technique especially effective, and cavity strike is often used immediately thereafter.

Downing the Enemy (Shuai Jiao, 摔跤)
Downing the enemy techniques destroy the opponent's balance and either cause him to fall or bounce him away. This category includes trips, takedowns, and throws, as well as pushes. To down the opponent, you must first be able to sense his jing; then you must understand his weighting and where his center of mass is, as well as the direction in which he is most easily uprooted. You can either use his jing against him or neutralize it and follow with techniques to make him lose his balance. To do these techniques effectively,

you must have a firm root. If you do not have a strong root, how can you destroy your opponent's root and make him fall? Second, you must be familiar with listening (ting, 聽), understanding (dong, 懂), neutralizing (hua, 化), leading (yin, 引), controlling (na, 拿), and rollback (lu, 掘) jing. Third, your body must be centered and move as a unit so that you can efficiently use your power.

Making the opponent fall is a fighting strategy used more for a friendly and/or unarmed opponent, and it is commonly used in pushing-hands competition. Another way to make the opponent fall is to use jing to bounce him away and force him to fall. This strategy is more offensive and is more likely to cause injury. In order to bounce the opponent, in addition to the above conditions you must also know several different kinds of emitting jin such as wardoff (peng, 掤), press (ji, 擠), and push (an, 按). It takes a long time to become skillful in these applications.

Qin Na (or Chin Na, 擒拿)

Qin na is a way to immobilize the opponent by controlling one or more of his joints. This joint control can be classified into two major strategies. One is called "misplacing the bones" (cuo gu, 錯骨), and the other is called "dividing the muscles" (fen jin, 分筋). Joints are connected with ligament and muscles. When a joint is bent at an abnormal angle, the ligaments are torn where they connect to the bone, causing extreme pain. If bent beyond a certain limit, the joint will pop out (i.e., be misplaced). Also, when the joint is bent and twisted, the muscles in that area are overstressed, which also causes significant pain. After a certain point, the muscle tissue will be divided and damaged.

Qin na control plays an important role in taijiquan. These techniques are usually applied immediately after the opponent's jing is neutralized. Qin na techniques are also commonly used in pushing-hands competition. For more qin na theory, the reader should refer to the author's books *Analysis of Shaolin Chin Na*, 2nd edition; *Comprehensive Applications of Shaolin Chin Na*; and *Tai Chi Chin Na*, by YMAA Publication Center (www.ymaa.com).

Cavity Strike (Dian Xue, 點穴)

Cavity strike is an attacking method in which a martial artist uses his jing or qi to strike the opponent's acupuncture cavities in order to control or kill him. In the human body there are 108 acupuncture cavities (out of more than 700 available) that can be used for martial purposes. When struck, 36 of these 108 cavities can be fatal, and the remaining 72 can cause numbness, fainting, or pain. Some of these cavities, when struck, will cause the breath to be sealed. Others will close an artery and affect the transportation of blood and oxygen to the brain. The others, when struck, can cause organ failure and even death. In order to make the cavity strike effective, the jing or qi must be strong, the strike must be accurate, and the time of striking must be right. This is the highest level of martial arts. Because of the killing potential of cavity strikes, this category is usually forbidden in pushing-hands or taijiquan free-fighting competition.

In addition to acupuncture cavities, organs are also targeted. The most common targets are the eyes, liver, and kidneys.

2-3. Analysis of Taijiquan Techniques

In this section we will analyze each form in the taijiquan sequence and discuss some of the possible martial applications. It is our hope that the reader develops an understanding of how to analyze techniques. Understanding how to analyze techniques is the trick that turns the rock into gold, which is preferable to just obtaining the gold itself. There are many possible applications for each form, and it is almost impossible to list every one of them. As your taijiquan knowledge and ability increase, your ability to analyze will also increase. For this reason, your application of a form might be different over a period of time. If you study this book and discuss every aspect with your training partners, you will learn how to analyze techniques and will have the chance to eventually master taijiquan applications.

Many of the applications of the forms have been hidden in the names of the forms. An example is pick up needle from sea bottom (hai di lao zhen, 海底撈針). In Chinese, the perineum is called the sea bottom (hai di, 海底), and a main application of the form is to attack the groin. In order to help you catch these hidden and implied applications, we will translate the Chinese name of each form before analyzing the applications. Many of the common translations of names of forms do not match the original Chinese meaning. Also, in some cases, the meaning of a name is obscure. This may be due to changes brought about by centuries of oral transmission, where discrepancies have arisen due to such factors as limited understanding and differences in dialects.

There are many styles of taijiquan. After so many hundreds of years of teaching and research, many different concepts, ideas, and understandings have evolved. For this reason, even though different styles may have similar forms with similar names, the applications may not be the same. Despite this, however, they must all follow the same general rules and principles; otherwise, the techniques would not be effective.

The reader should also understand that the taijiquan sequence does not contain all the taijiquan martial techniques. The techniques in the sequence only serve as an introduction to help the practitioner understand the foundation and principles. After you understand all these applications, you should then study more advanced techniques from pushing hands and the two-person fighting set. In this section, we will use the forms from the long Yang style that has low stances and large postures. Each posture will be briefly described before the techniques are discussed. For details and continuity, please refer to the author's taijiquan books and DVDs by YMAA Publication Center (www.ymaa.com).

Yang-Style Taijiquan Techniques

1. Grasp Sparrow's Tail: Right and Left (Lan Que Wei, 攬雀尾)

Grasp sparrow's tail in Chinese is lan que wei. Lan means grasp or seize. This implies that when you apply this technique, you not only intercept your opponent's strike but also grasp him. A sparrow's tail is very light and fragile, and also sensitive and mobile. Therefore, when you grasp the sparrow's tail, you must be cautious and sensitive, and you cannot use muscular strength. You must lead your enemy's attack lightly and skillful into a bad position where you can do the technique. In the taijiquan sequence, there are two forms of grasp sparrow's tail: right and left. However, the left form should be the follow-up to the right form, and so some taijiquan masters would prefer to refer to the left grasp sparrow's tail as diagonal flying (left).

Movements:

To do grasp sparrow's tail to the right, move your right hand upward, with your left hand near the inside of your right elbow, and at the same time move your left leg close to the right with just the toes of the left foot touching the ground. To do the left side, step your left leg backward and turn your body left so that you face to the rear in a mountain-climbing stance. As you turn your body, your right hand moves down and your left hand moves up.

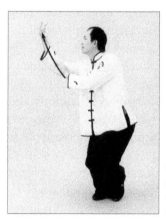

Grasp sparrow's tail: right (you lan que wei).

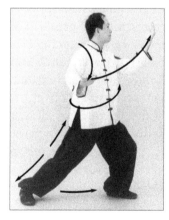

Grasp sparrow's tail: left (zuo lan que wei), also known as diagonal flying left.

Analysis:

Your right hand moves up to intercept the opponent's punch and lift it upward, exposing his chest to your attack. Your left hand is ready to protect your chest or control his elbow. Moving the left leg close to the right leg during deflection closes your groin area and protects the groin from a kick. Only the toes of the left foot touch the ground, and there is no weight on it, which allows you to kick anytime you want. Grasp sparrow's tail: right deflects the opponent's punch and also sets him up for your attack. In the sequence, the left form is done in the opposite direction, though in an actual application it would be done facing the same direction. For example, you can step back if your opponent continues his attack, or you can step forward to attack, using your left leg to block the opponent's leg and prevent his retreat. There are two keys to making this technique effective. First, after your right hand has intercepted the opponent's punch, you must immediately grab his arm. Second, when your left hand raises up to attack, your right hand must move down to balance your jing.

Downing the Enemy

Application 1

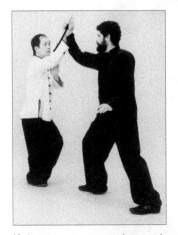 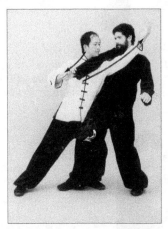 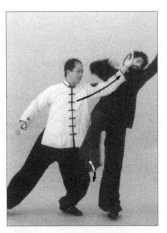

If the opponent punches with his right hand, deflect his arm upward.

Turn down your right hand to control his wrist as you step your left leg behind his right leg.

Next use wardoff jing (peng, 掤) with your left arm to the side to make him fall.

The trick to making your opponent fall is to execute wardoff sideways with your left arm and at the same time push the opponent's right thigh with your left thigh in order to break his root.

Application 2

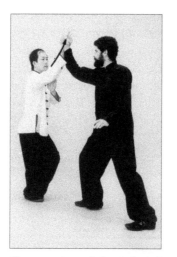
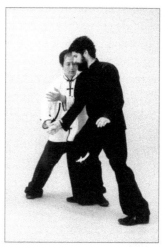

Once you have deflected your opponent's arm upward, you can then pluck down and at the same time step your left leg behind his right leg, placing your left thigh close to or touching his right thigh.

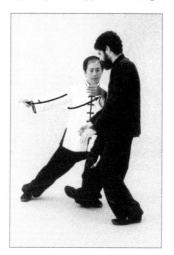
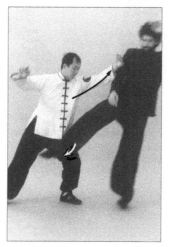

At the same time, place your left arm against his right arm to immobilize it.

When all of this is set up, use your wardoff jing to bounce him away or make him fall.

Application 3

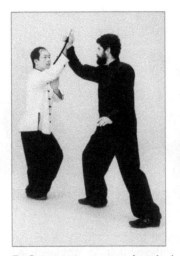 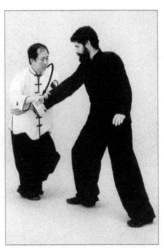

Deflect your opponent's right-hand attack, upward, and then pluck it down.

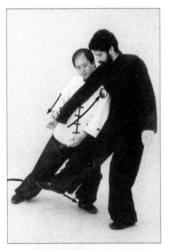 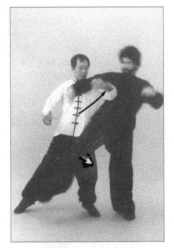

Step your left leg behind his right leg, with your thigh touching his thigh to prevent him from stepping backward.

Next hit or push him with your shoulder under his armpit.

Application 4

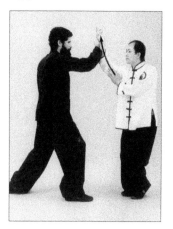 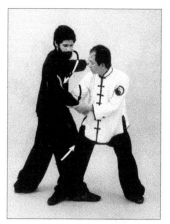 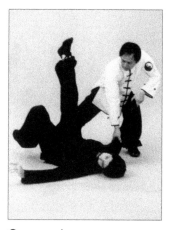

Deflect your opponent's right-hand attack, upward.

Pluck his arm down and grasp his wrist with your left hand, and slide your right hand toward his elbow. While you are doing this, place your left foot on the floor and then step your right foot behind his right foot, with your thigh touching his thigh.

Once you have your opponent in this position, immediately pull his arm down and at the same time bounce your thigh back to make him fall.

Qin Na Control

Application 1

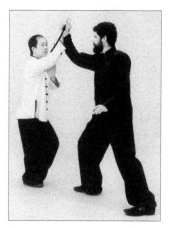 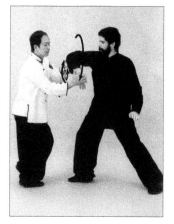

Deflect your opponent's attack, upward.

Next turn down your right hand to grasp his wrist, and at the same time control his elbow with your left hand.

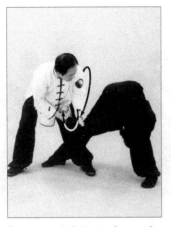

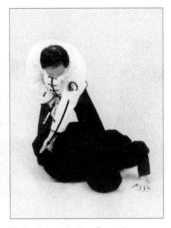

Step your left leg in front of his right leg, with the back of your thigh touching his knee or thigh, and push his elbow forward as you pull his hand backward.

Take him to the floor by pulling him forward as you slide your left foot backward. This is a combination of qin na control and downing the enemy.

Application 2

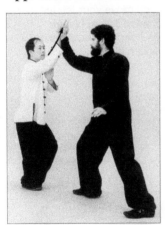

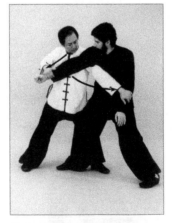

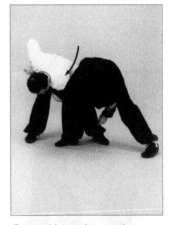

Deflect your opponent's right punch, upward.

Grasp his wrist with your right hand and pull downward, and at the same time step your left foot behind his right leg. While you are doing this, also place your left arm under his armpit and control his body and left arm.

Control his right arm by holding it tight across your chest. Once you have set up this position, bow forward and use your left shoulder to press down the back of the opponent's shoulder.

Application 3

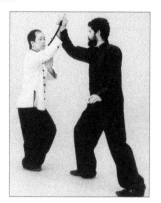

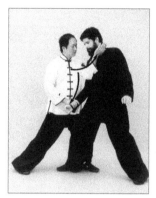

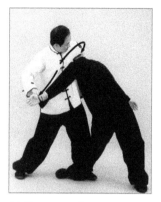

Deflect the opponent's right punch, upward.

Grasp his right wrist and pull it down as you step your left leg behind his right leg.

At the same time, move your left hand toward his neck and circle backward to hold his neck.

As in the last technique, use your chest to control the opponent's elbow and immobilize his right arm. If you move your left leg forward as you pull his head back, you can easily make him fall.

Application 4

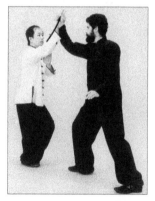

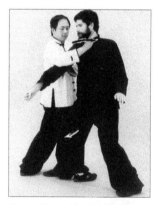

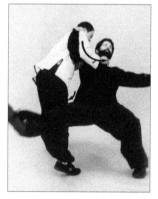

Deflect the opponent's punch, upward.

Grasp his right wrist and pull down as you grasp his right elbow with your left hand. Then step your right leg behind his right leg, and at the same time slide your right hand up to his throat.

Once you have set up this position, bounce your thigh backward to break the opponent's root and push your right hand downward to bring him to the ground. This is a combination of qin na control and downing the enemy.

Application 5

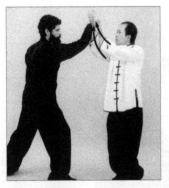 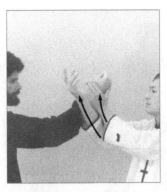

When you deflect your opponent's attack upward, slide your left hand up along your right arm and grasp his right hand.

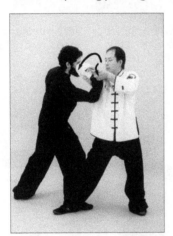 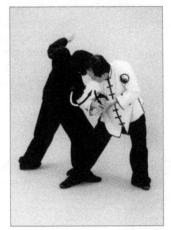

Next circle your right elbow over and behind his arm and down to lock his elbow, and then up to lock both his wrist and elbow. You can also sweep your right leg backward to make him fall.

Cavity Strike or Striking the Vital Points

This category of applications can actually be easier than the other two. Usually downing the enemy and qin na control take longer to apply than a strike, and so your enemy has more time to sense and react to your attack. If you can apply these two categories of applications easily, you should have little difficulty with striking because there are so many important targets. However, striking acupuncture cavities is considerably more difficult than hitting organs or other vital areas. First, you must know the correct location and depth of the cavities you wish to strike. Second, you must know the time of day when the cavities are vulnerable. Because cavity strikes can easily hurt or kill people, the locations and vulnerable times of the cavities are usually kept secret. Here we will show some of the possible strikes.

Application 1

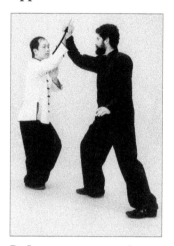

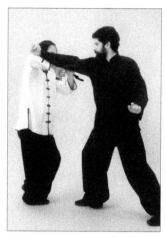

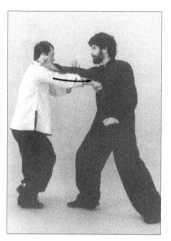

Deflect your opponent's attack, upward.

Seal his elbow with your left hand to block further action, then slide your right hand under his arm.

You can then strike the opponent's chest with your fist.

Application 2

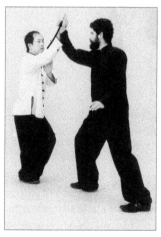

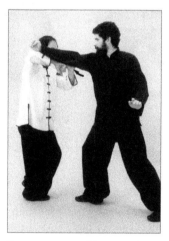

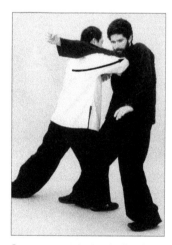

Deflect your opponent's attack, upward.

Set up your striking position by sealing your opponent's elbow with your left hand to block further action.

Step your right leg behind the opponent's right leg and at the same time strike with your elbow.

Application 3

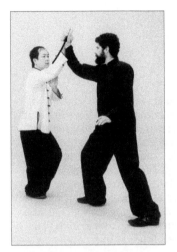

Deflect your opponent's
attack.

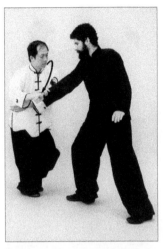

Seal his elbow with your left
hand to block further attack.

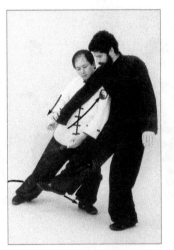

Step your left leg behind his
right leg, with your thigh
touching his thigh to prevent
him from stepping backward.

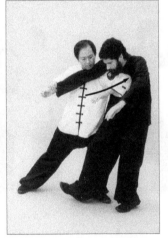

Use your elbow to strike his
chest.

Application 4

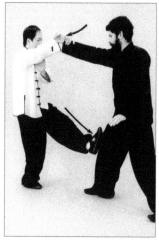

In grasp sparrow's tail: right, only the toes of your left foot touch the floor, so your left leg is alive and can be used for sudden attacks. In this application, after you have deflected the opponent's attack, grasp his right wrist with your right hand and step kick his right knee with your left foot.

Application 5

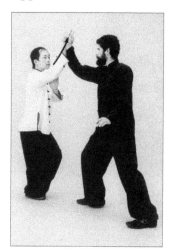

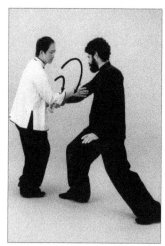

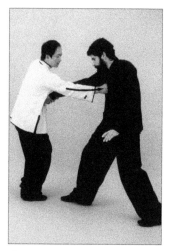

Deflect your opponent's strike.

Stick to his arm and circle it downward to expose his chest.

Control his right hand with your left hand, and strike his chest with your right fist.

2. Wardoff (Peng, 掤)

The Chinese word for wardoff is peng. Peng means to arc your arms and use them to push or bounce something away. It is used in expressions like peng kai (掤 開) (push open or push away), which refers to the motion you would use to wade through a crowd and bounce people out of your way. In taijiquan, anytime you use your arm to push someone or something away, it is called peng.

In the taijiquan sequence, you prepare for peng by rotating your body to the left, drawing your right leg in, next to the left leg with the toes of the right foot touching the floor, and raising your left arm and lowering your right arm so they look as if you are holding a large ball. Then you step back with your right leg, turn on the heels one at a time toward the opposite direction, and rotate your body forward, raising your right arm and lowering your left. In the applications you will not turn to the opposite direction.

Movements:

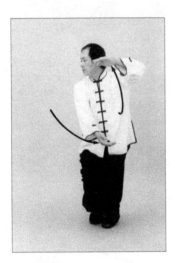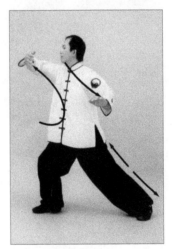

Analysis:

You can use your left forearm to intercept the opponent's left or right punch. After you deflect, your enemy's chest will be exposed for your strike. You can also use your left arm to deflect the opponent's attack and lead him into an unbalanced position, and then bounce him away with your right arm. When your right leg moves close to your left leg, it protects the groin from attack, and is also set up for kicking. When you use peng to bounce your enemy, treat yourself like a beach ball bouncing an outside pressure away. Also, when you bounce, your direction should be forward and slightly upward to pull the enemy's root up so that he will move more easily.

Downing the Enemy

Application 1

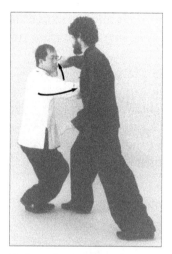 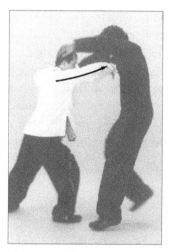

Deflect the opponent's right-hand strike with your left hand.

Next step forward with your right leg and use your right forearm to bounce away the opponent.

Application 2

The same application can also be used if your opponent strikes with his left hand.

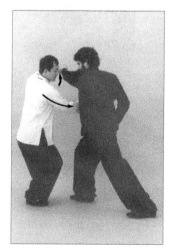 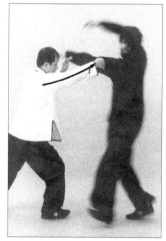

Deflect the left-hand strike with your left hand.

Next step forward to bounce him away.

Application 3

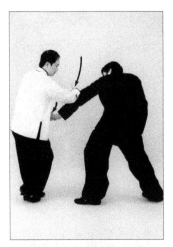

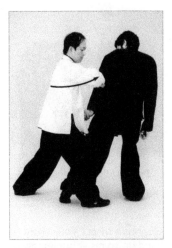

Deflect the opponent's left-handed attack. Grasp his wrist and pull it down. Use your right forearm to press down on his elbow.

If your opponent attempts to pull back from your grasp, follow his motion and use your right forearm to bounce him away.

Application 4

Qin na techniques are often used in coordination with downing the enemy or cavity-strike techniques to increase their effectiveness.

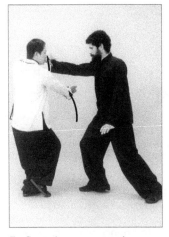

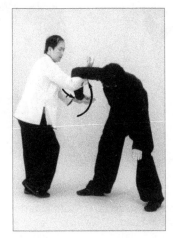

Deflect the opponent's punch with your left hand.

Lock his elbow with your right hand.

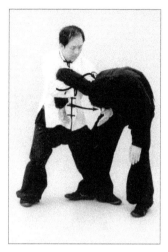 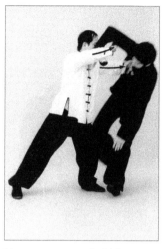

Continue to coil your right hand up to his shoulder, and place your left forearm on his side.

Use your control of his arm to bend him forward, and when he resists and tries to pull back, use left wardoff to bounce him away.

Qin Na Control

Application 1

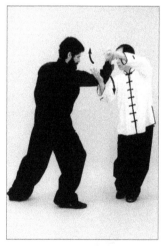 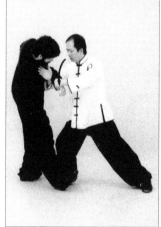

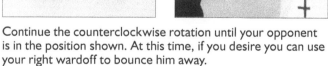

Deflect the opponent's right punch with your left hand, place your right hand under his elbow and rotate both your hands counterclockwise.

Continue the counterclockwise rotation until your opponent is in the position shown. At this time, if you desire you can use your right wardoff to bounce him away.

Application 2

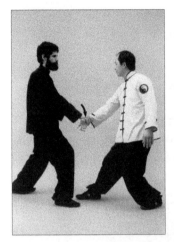 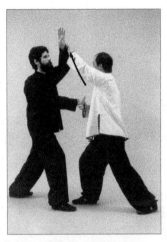 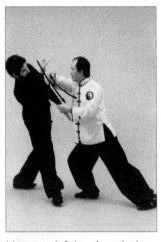

Your opponent grasps your right wrist with his right hand.

Fake an attack to his eyes with your left hand. Your opponent will naturally block with his left hand to protect his eyes.

Use your left hand to pluck his left arm downward over his right arm, and raise your right arm and execute wardoff to lock both his arms.

Cavity Strike or Striking the Vital Points

All the applications shown above can be used as a strike. However, when wardoff is used for striking, a shorter jing is used. There is an additional application that is set up in the sequence but not actually done. When you deflect in the beginning of wardoff, your right foot touches the ground with the toes only. Your weight is off the foot and it can easily kick.

Application 1

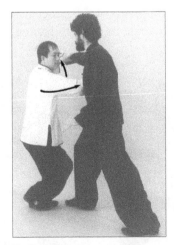 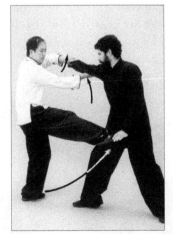

Deflect your opponent's strike.

Use your right foot to kick the opponent's groin.

3. Rollback (Lu, 擴)

Rollback in Chinese is called lu. Lu means to rotate, lead, or pull. It is commonly used in expressions like lu kai (擴開) (to pull open) or lu dao (擴倒) (to pull down).

Movements:

In the taijiquan sequence, rollback has two major applications: small rollback (xiao lu, 小擴) and large rollback (da lu, 大擴).

Small Rollback. First lift your right forearm up and circle your hand clockwise. Then, with your elbow down, shift your weight to the rear and sit on your rear leg in a four-six stance (si liu bu, 四六步), while turning your body so that your arms draw back slightly to your left.

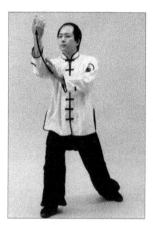 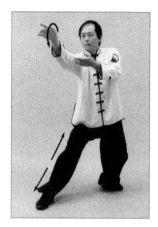

Large Rollback. Circle your right hand, then shift your weight to the rear and sit on your rear leg in a four-six stance, while turning your body to draw your hand back with the elbow down toward your left side. The main points of difference between this move and small rollback are that the lead hand can circle in either direction, you sit back a little further, and you turn your body more.

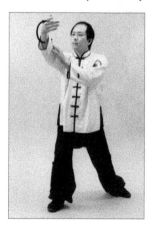 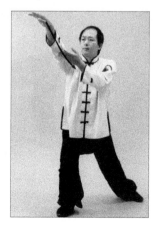 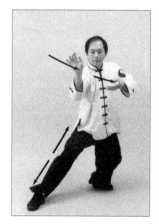

Analysis:

The first part of this form is used to intercept and connect to the opponent's arm. Once you have connected, you then execute rollback to lead his force sideward and past you. When you do small rollback, the movements are small and quick with the intent of exposing your opponent's vital cavities to attack. Large rollback is a larger move that is commonly used to pull the opponent's center and make him lose balance so that you can attack. It is frequently used with a step backward. In order for your rollback to be effective, you must have a firm root and good listening, understanding, adhering and sticking, and leading jing.

Downing the Enemy: Small Rollback

Application 1

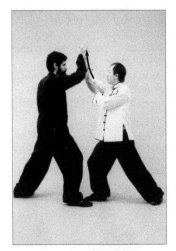
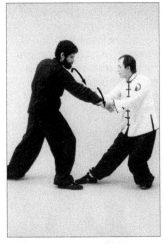

Use your forearm to intercept your opponent's attack.

After you connect, immediately execute rollback and lead his arm back and to your side.

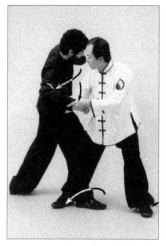 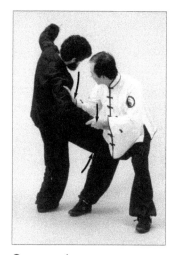

If you pull strongly to your left, you can make your opponent lose his balance. Alternatively, right after your rollback, immediately hop your rear leg forward and place your right leg behind the opponent's right leg.

Once you have set up this position, pull his arm sideward and downward and at the same time bounce your knee or thigh backward to uproot the opponent's front foot and make him fall.

Application 2

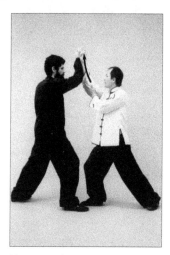 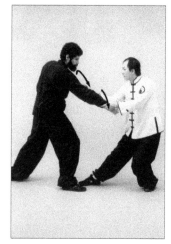

Use your forearm to intercept your opponent's attack. Execute rollback to your left.

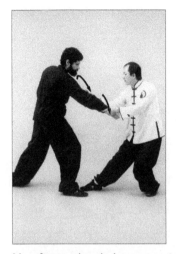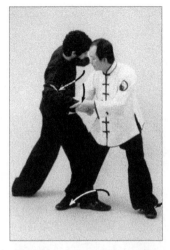

Hop forward and place your right leg behind the opponent's right leg.

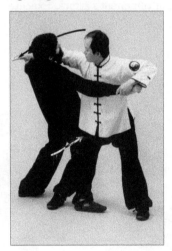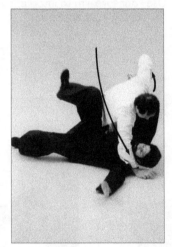

Circle your right arm around his neck and press him down.

Application 3

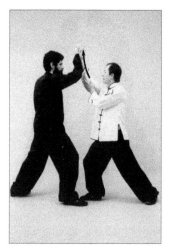 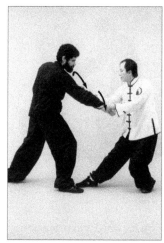

Use your forearm to intercept your opponent's attack. Execute rollback to your left.

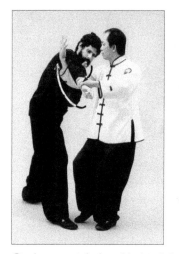 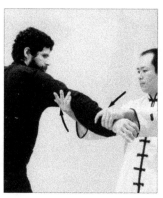 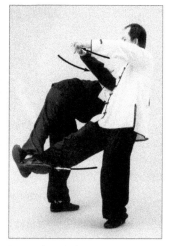

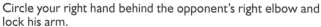

Circle your right hand behind the opponent's right elbow and lock his arm.

Immediately hop your rear leg forward and use your front leg to sweep his right leg and make him fall.

Qin Na Control: Small Rollback

Application 1

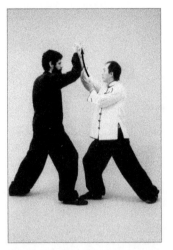 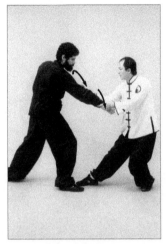

Use your forearm to intercept your opponent's attack.
Execute rollback to your left.

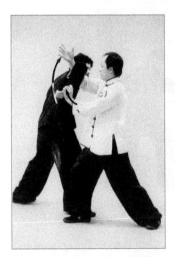 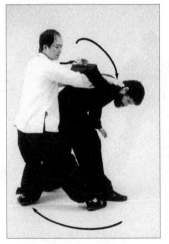 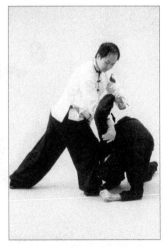

Circle your right arm and step your right leg behind the opponent's right leg. Your left hand should control his right wrist.

Continue the motion by stepping your left leg behind him, and place your right hand on his shoulder.

Shift your weight forward and press down with both hands.

Cavity Strike or Striking the Vital Points: Small Rollback

Application 1

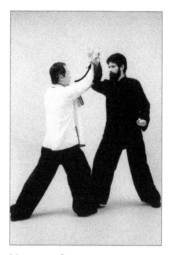 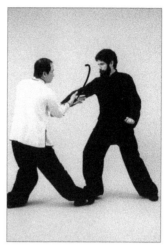

Use your forearm to intercept your opponent's attack.
Execute rollback to your left.

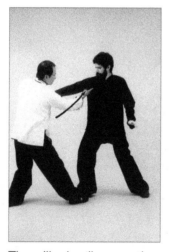 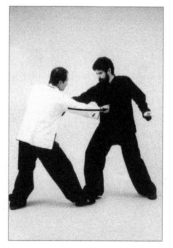

The rollback will expose the
front of your opponent's
body. You can strike his
armpit.

You can also target his solar
plexus, throat, or other vital
cavities.

Application 2

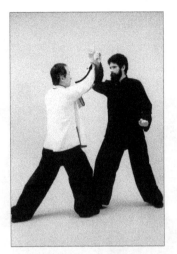 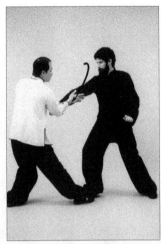

Use your forearm to intercept your opponent's attack.
Execute rollback to your left.

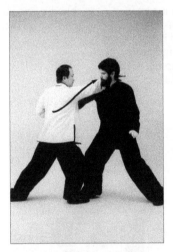 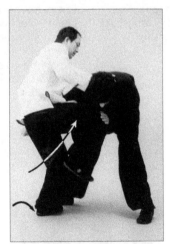

Slide your right hand up your
opponent's right arm and
hook his neck.

Immediately hop forward
and use your right knee to
kick his chest or face while
your right hand presses
downward.

Downing the Enemy: Large Rollback

Application 1

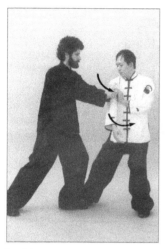

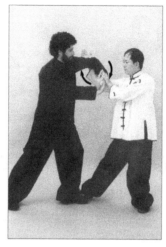

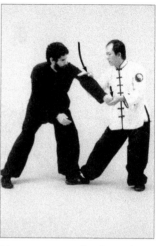

Yield to your opponent's punch or push by sitting back to lead his power into emptiness.

Rotate your right arm counterclockwise so that your right hand is just above his left elbow, and at the same time grasp his left wrist with your left hand.

Next turn your body to draw him off balance to his front.

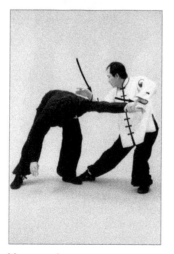

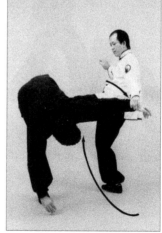

You now have your opponent in a bad situation. You can pull with your left hand and push with your right and make him lose his balance.

To worsen his situation, you can add a leg sweep with your left leg and make him fall.

Application 2

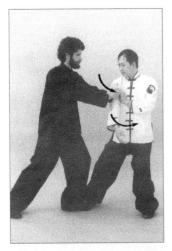 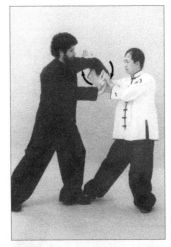 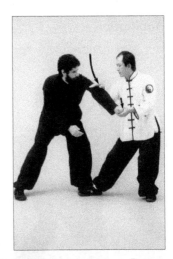

Yield to your opponent's punch or push by sitting back to lead his power into emptiness. Rotate your right arm counterclockwise so that your right hand is just above his left elbow, and at the same time grasp his left wrist with your left hand. Execute rollback to your left.

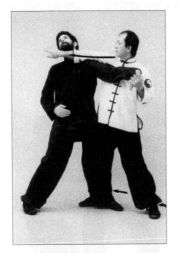 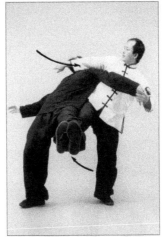

Immediately hop forward and place you right leg behind your opponent's left leg and simultaneously slide your right arm up his left arm to his neck.

Sweep with your right leg and at the same time press your right arm downward to make him fall.

Qin Na Control: Large Rollback

Application 1

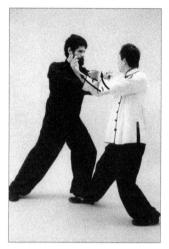 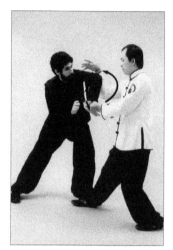 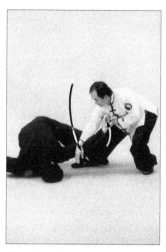

When the opponent presses your chest, sit back to yield and use your right arm and left hand to connect to him.

Next circle both hands to control his wrist and elbow.

Continue this rotation and drop your body until your opponent's face reaches the floor.

Application 2

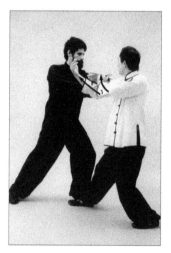 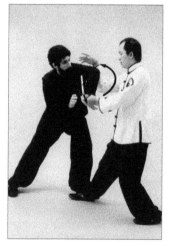

When the opponent presses your chest, sit back to yield and use your right arm and left hand to connect to him. Next circle both hands to control his wrist and elbow.

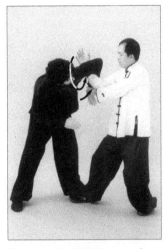

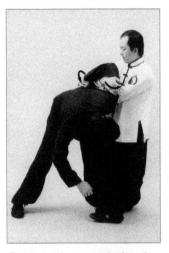

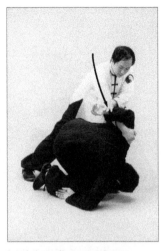

Continue circling your right arm around his arm.

Circle until your right hand reaches his shoulder.

Lock his elbow and press your right hand down until his face reaches the floor.

Application 3

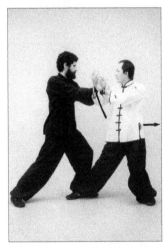

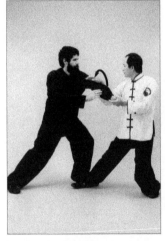

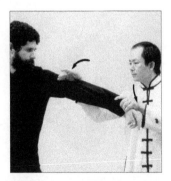

Yield from your opponent's attack into a large rollback.

Keep your opponent's arm straight.

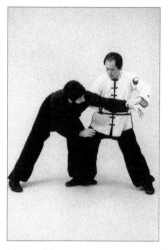
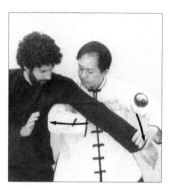
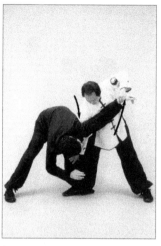

Next slide your upper arm to his shoulder.

Press downward with your right upper arm as you pull upward with your left hand.

Cavity Strike or Striking the Vital Points: Large Rollback

Application 1

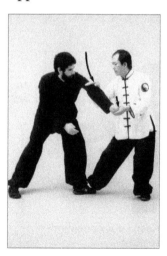
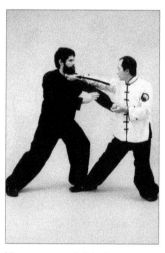
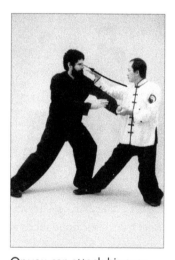

Your rollback may open your opponent's face to attack.

You can attack his throat.

Or you can attack his eyes.

Application 2

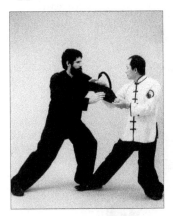 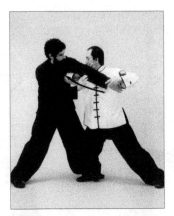 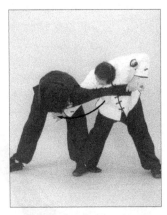

Your rollback may expose the area under your opponent's armpit to attack.

You may then use your elbow to strike the exposed cavities.

Alternatively, you can extend your hand to hit or grab his groin.

Application 3

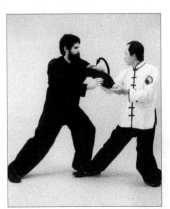 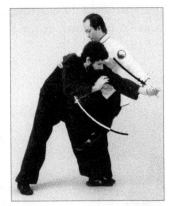

Apply large rollback.

Next you can pull his left hand to your rear and at the same time use your knee to kick his abdomen.

4. Press (Ji, 擠)

The Chinese word for this form is ji, and it means to squeeze or press against. Both hands are used to press against your opponent or to squeeze part of his body. The character for ji is made up of two figures meaning "hand" and "even," and has the meaning of using your hands to even something off. This is sometimes reflected in pushing hands, when you feel some part of the opponent suddenly become substantial and you press that spot back.

Movements:

After you execute rollback, use the left hand on the right wrist to press forward.

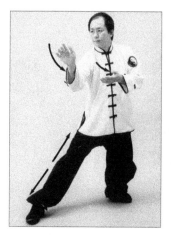 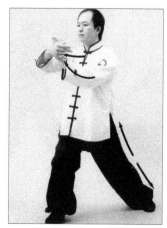

Analysis:

This form is commonly used for long jing, even though the attacking movement is short. The main purpose of this form is to make the opponent fall or bounce away, although it is also used to strike areas such as the solar plexus to seal the breath, or the shoulder blade to numb the shoulder.

Downing the Enemy

Application 1

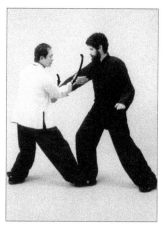 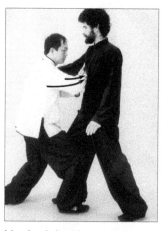 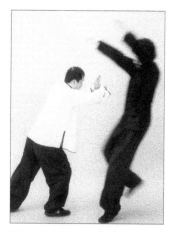

Execute rollback with your opponent's right arm.

Use both hands to press against the opponent's chest at the solar plexus.

When you press forward, your front thigh should bounce to the left to affect the opponent's front root so that he can be more easily uprooted.

At this point, you should understand the reason that a person can be bounced away if his solar plexus area is pressed or pushed. If you check an anatomy book, you will see the rib cage is not a continuous piece of bone. It is made of sections that are connected by strong ligaments. It protects the vital organs in your chest from outside blows, so when there is an outside attack that is strong enough to damage the organs, the chest behaves like a spring or ball and either bounces the attack away or else bounces you

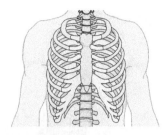

Rib cage.

away from the attack. Therefore, if you have a firm root and apply a strong push onto the opponent's solar plexus area, his ribs will give and then spring back, bouncing him away from you. If the rib cage was not constructed in pieces connected by ligaments, but instead was made of single pieces of bone, a strong attack would easily break it and injure the organs.

Sometimes you may see martial artists demonstrate their power by striking someone's solar plexus or chest area and bouncing them several yards away. You should understand that as long as you have a firm root and enough press jing, you could do the same thing. However, you should also understand that it is an immoral demonstration, because in order to make someone bounce himself away like this, your power has to be strong enough to damage his organs, especially his heart. The demonstration may be impressive, but you will be inflicting internal damage on your partner.

Application 2

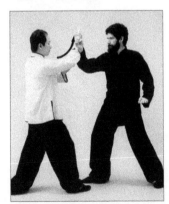

Intercept your opponent's strike with your right hand.

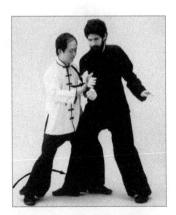

Guide his right hand down and place both your hands on his upper arm. Step your left leg behind his right leg to put him in an awkward position.

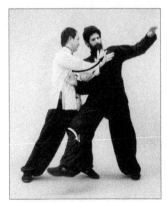

Emit your force to your left front, against his chest. At the same time, bounce your left thigh to the right to uproot his right foot.

Application 3

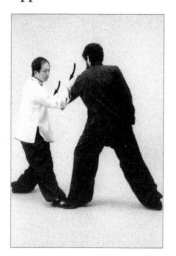 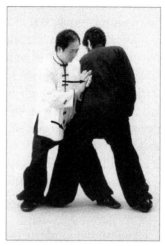 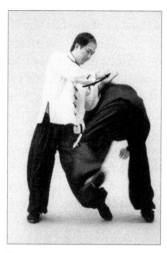

| Your opponent strikes with his left hand and with his left leg forward. Apply large rollback. | Step forward and place both hands on the back of your opponent's side, with your leg locking the opponent's front leg. | Press your hands to the side and use your thigh to destroy the opponent's front root. |

Application 4

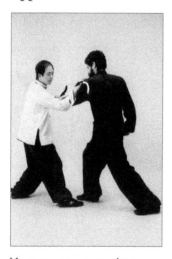 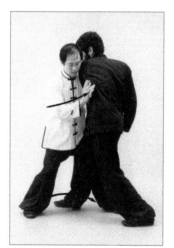 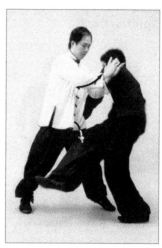

Your opponent punches with his left hand and steps forward with his right foot.

Step forward and place both hands on the back of your opponent's side, with your leg locking the opponent's front leg. Press your hands to the side and use your thigh to destroy the opponent's front root.

Qin Na Control

Application 1

When press is used in qin na techniques, both hands are squeezed together to lock a joint such as the wrist.

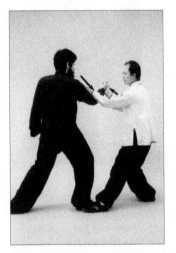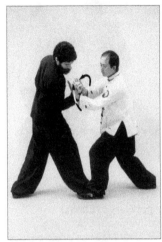

Forward squeeze used to lock the wrist.

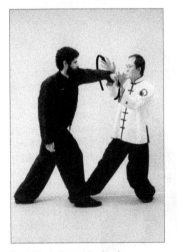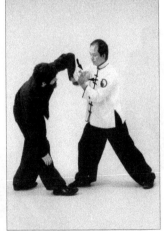

Reverse squeeze lock.

Cavity Strike or Striking the Vital Points

Application 1

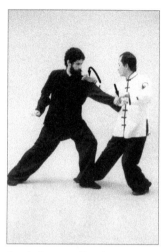 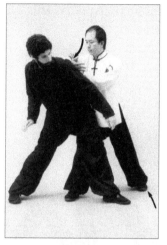

Apply large rollback to put your opponent in a disadvantageous position.

Readjust your legs and use both hands to press strike the shoulder blade.

Application 2

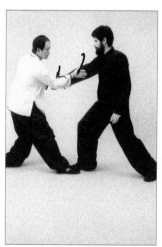 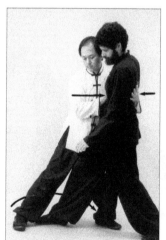

Apply small rollback to neutralize the opponent's attack.

Step your left leg behind the opponent's right leg. At the same time, place your right hand on the opponent's solar plexus and your left hand on his back. You can then squeeze both hands together to shock the opponent's heart or seal his breath. When you place your hands this way, your opponent's self-protecting rib structure will not be able to effectively protect him from your attack.

Application 3

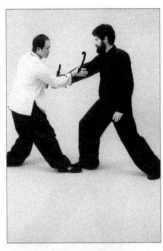

Apply small rollback to neutralize the opponent's attack.

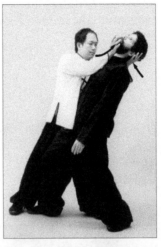

Place your right hand on his chin or neck and your left hand behind his head. If you jerk your power upward, you could knock him out. If you twist both hands to the side, you could break his neck.

5. Push (An, 按)

The Chinese word for this form is *an*. The Chinese character for the word is made up of two figures meaning "hand" (扌) and "peace" (安) and has the meaning of using your hands to hold someone down and inhibit his motion. In everyday speech, *an* means to press or push down. In taijiquan, *an* can be used for either offense or defense. When it is used for offense, it is used to push and bounce the opponent away or to push strike the vital cavities. When it is used for defense, it is used to stick to the opponent's arm and immobilize it, preventing further action. When it is applied onto your enemy, he should feel that his arms have been pressed down and he can neither lift them up nor get away. In offense, push can be used in any direction. When it is used for defense, it is usually directed downward.

Movements:

The hands are usually first drawn in toward the chest to accumulate energy, and then stretched out as you emit. The motion is either forward or downward.

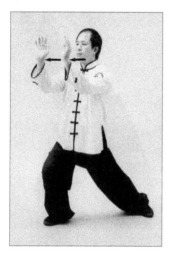 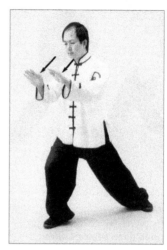

Analysis:

Like press, push is mainly used as a long jing, although it is sometimes used with short jing for cavity strikes. To understand how to use push jing (or press jing) to bounce the opponent, imagine that you are pushing a large beach ball and trying to bounce it away. If your jing is too short, the ball will bounce you away. However, if your jing is long and you have a good root, then the energy that the ball accumulates will bounce it away.

In taijiquan, when you want to uproot the opponent and bounce him away, you should push forward and upward. When you want to make your opponent lose his stability and fall, you should push to the side or downward. To strike the opponent in the stomach or immobilize his arms, push downward. You can use a single hand push to strike the opponent's solar plexus and bounce him away by using the same principle that was explained in the discussion of press. Naturally, in order to generate enough power to bounce or uproot your opponent, you must have a firm root first and then you must have strong push jing.

Downing the Enemy

Application 1

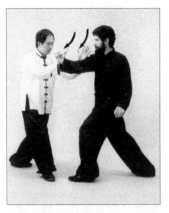 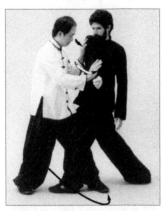 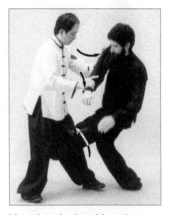

Your opponent punches with his right hand with his left leg forward. Neutralize his power to the side.

Next step your left leg to the outside of his left leg.

Your hands should push downward to immobilize your opponent as you step in. Once you are in position, use your right hand to pull him into an unbalanced position and your left hand to push him sideward. In order to destroy your opponent's front root, your left thigh should bounce back while your hands are pushing.

Application 2

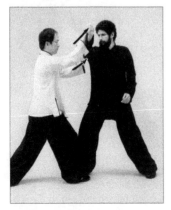 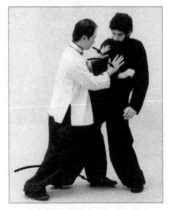 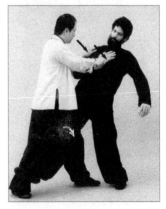

Your opponent punches you with his right hand with his right leg forward. Neutralize his punch to the right.

Immediately push down on his arm with both hands to seal him and prevent further action as you step behind his right leg with your left leg to stop him from retreating.

Once this position is set up, push forward and downward while pushing his thigh with your leg.

Application 3

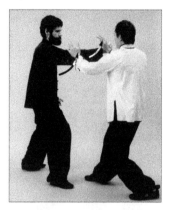

Neutralize your opponent's punch to the right.

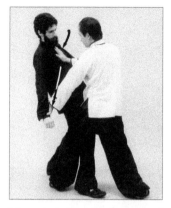

Next circle his arm downward and to the side to open his chest while your left leg steps behind his right leg to prevent his retreat.

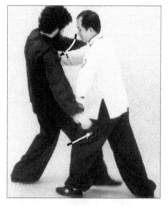

Once you have put your opponent in this position, push down with your right hand and at the same time bounce your left thigh against his right leg to uproot his front foot. In this application, because your right hand can easily reach his chest, you can apply short push jing to strike a cavity to seal his breath or even kill him.

Application 4

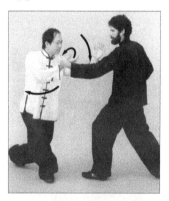

Your opponent punches with his left hand while his left leg is forward. Neutralize his punch to your right.

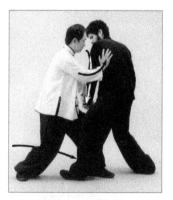

Next continue circling his arm downward and to the other side. At the same time, step your left leg forward inside his left leg, and place your right hand on his shoulder blade.

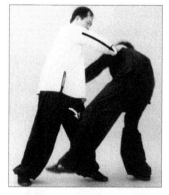

Immediately push forward and to the side with your right hand as you bounce your left thigh against his front thigh to destroy his root. Because your right hand is on your opponent's shoulder blade, you can use short push jing to strike the center of his shoulder blade to numb the shoulder.

Cavity Strike or Striking the Vital Points

Application 1

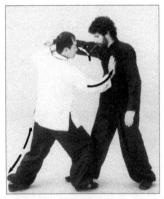 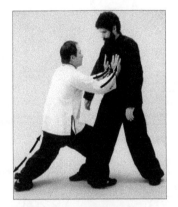

If you can reach your opponent's chest with one or both hands, you can use a hand to strike his solar plexus.

If long push jing is used, you may bounce the opponent away, but if short pushing jing is used, you could shock his heart or break his ribs and kill him. Similarly, you can use short jing to strike the chest (nipple area) with both hands to seal the opponent's breath. Alternatively, you can use long jing to push the bottom ribs to bounce him away. In order to make all these applications effective, your jing should be directed forward and upward.

Application 2

Downward push jing is a kind of sinking jing that is often used to strike the stomach area to seal the breath. To seal the opponent's breath, you can grasp the opponent's throat to stop him from taking air into his lung, or you can strike an area that will cause his lungs to contract and he will be unable to take in any air. The first kind of sealing the breath is obvious and clear; therefore, we will not discuss it further here. When the second kind of sealing the breath is used, you must make the muscles around the lungs contract in order to compress the lungs. There are muscles on the outside of the ribs, but striking these muscles will only cause pain and perhaps some internal bruising—it will not cause the lung to constrict. To seal the breath, you must make the muscles inside the rib cage contract. To make the muscles contract, you need to know the spots where certain nerve endings or qi channels that are connected to the internal muscles are exposed outside of the ribs.

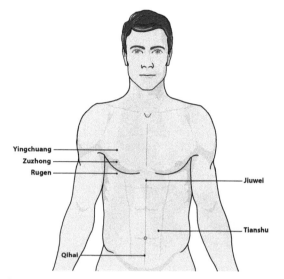

Exposed cavities.

When these cavities are properly struck, the qi will be disturbed and will shock the internal muscles into contracting, which will compress the lungs. Alternatively, you can strike certain areas or cavities below the rib cage where the muscles that surround the lungs extend. When these areas are struck, the muscles will contract and compress the lungs. Usually, striking cavities on the chest is harder to do correctly than striking the stomach area, but it can be more effective. It requires great accuracy and knowledge of the depth of the cavities, but the shock is directly to the lungs.

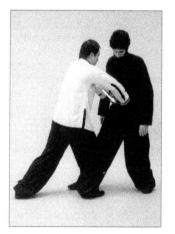 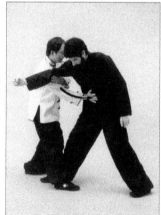

Examples of double- and single-handed attacks to the stomach area to seal the opponent's breath.

6. Single Whip (Dan Bian, 單鞭)

The name refers to the way the right hand is held in the sequence; the movement of the left hand is a follow-up movement. The Chinese name is dan bian. Dan means single or alone. Bian is a whip that can be made of leather, rattan, or even wood. When it is made of leather, it is call ruan bian (軟鞭), or soft whip. When it is made of rattan, it is called ruan ying bian (軟硬鞭), which means soft-hard whip. When it is made of wood, it is called ying bian (硬鞭), which means hard whip. In ancient times a whip was necessary when riding a horse, and naturally techniques were developed for using the whip in battle. Because the whip is not sharp, it is usually only used for deflecting.

In taijiquan, single whip is used to lead the opponent's hand or weapon past your body. The motion is similar to how you might use the whip when riding a horse. The deflection can be soft like a soft whip or hard like a hard whip, depending on the situation.

Movements:

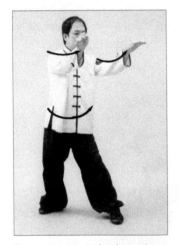
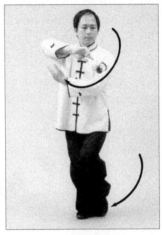
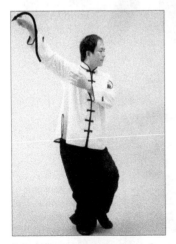

First rotate your body to the left with your hands in front of you and the elbows sunken.

Turn your body to the right as you continue to circle your left hand down to your stomach, while coiling your right hand upward and backward.

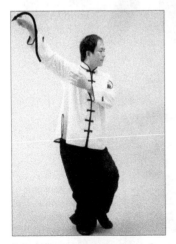
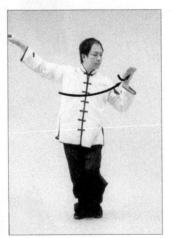
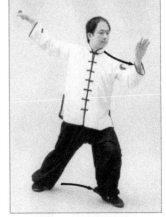

Rotate your body to the left and face forward as you block past your face with your left hand.

Twist your left hand to make your left palm face forward, then step forward and push.

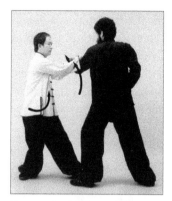

Rotate the body to deflect an attack to the side.

Analysis:

The rotation of the body to the left just before the whipping motion can be used to deflect an attack to the side. The whiplike motion of the right hand is used to lead the opponent's weapon or hand to the rear. The second half of the form is a follow-up form used for attack. Therefore, in the application, you first deflect the opponent's attack with your right hand, and then immediately use your left hand to continue the deflection, if necessary, and then strike. When you deflect, your left foot touches the floor with the toes only. This allows you to kick anytime the opportunity arises.

Downing the Enemy

Application 1

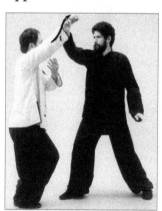

Deflect your opponent's punch to the right.

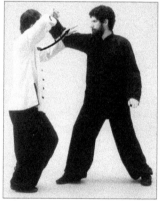

Use your left hand to move his hand to the side to expose his body.

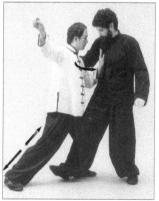

Next step your left leg behind his right leg.

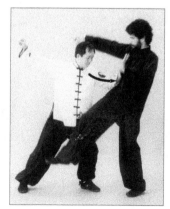

Push him away with your left hand while your left leg bounces against his right leg to destroy his root.

Qin Na Control

Application 1

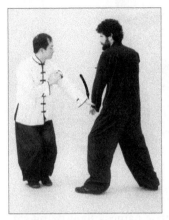 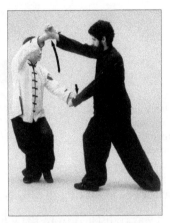 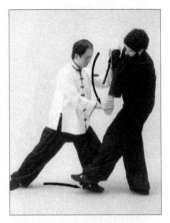

Grasp your opponent's left hand with your left hand and pull it down.

In this position your upper body is exposed, and that may lure the opponent into attacking your face with his right hand. If he does, use your right hand to deflect his attack and lead it to the right.

Immediately step your left leg inside his left leg and circle both your hands to lock his arms. As you can see, this application can also be used to bounce him away or make him fall.

Cavity Strike or Striking the Vital Points

Application 1

Using the same motions explained in the downing the enemy, application 1, use short push jing to strike the opponent's chest to seal his breath.

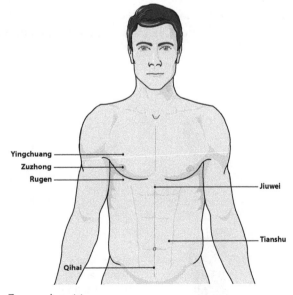

Yingchuang
Zuzhong
Rugen
Jiuwei
Tianshu
Qihai

Exposed cavities.

Application2

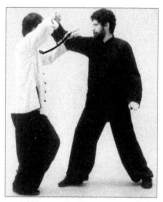

Use your left hand to move his hand to the side to expose his body.

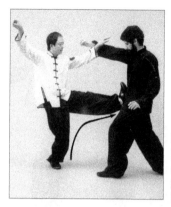

Use your left leg to kick the opponent's groin or dan tian (丹田).

7. Lift Hands and Lean Forward (Ti Shou Shang Shi, 提手上勢)

Lift hands and lean forward was translated from the Chinese name ti shou shang shi. Ti means to raise, pull up, or pick up. Therefore, ti shou means to raise your hands. Shang means up, and shi means posture. Therefore, the entire name should be translated as "raise hands to the up posture." Because many taijiquan books translated it as "lift hands and lean forward" or "lift hands and step forward," the author felt it was best to use the same name to avoid confusion. However, as an advanced taijiquan practitioner, you should know the exact meaning of the Chinese name. Remember that you should not lean your body forward or in any direction, because any leaning will make you lose your balance and center. Also, in the sequence, you do not really step forward but only move your leg forward to lightly touch the floor. Because there is no weight on this leg, it should not be called "step forward."

Movements:

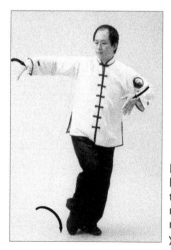

Lower your hands, and at the same time move your right leg near your left leg.

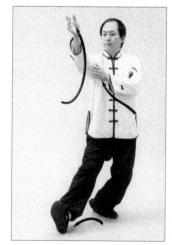

Continue the movement of your hands upward, in front of your chest, and simultaneously move your right leg forward and touch the floor with the heel.

Analysis:

When you lower both hands, you protect your dan tian area from attack. Bringing your right leg near the left leg seals your groin against kicks and hand attacks. When your opponent punches your upper body, raise your hands to lock his attack. Because your right leg is not rooted, it can be used for a quick kick.

Downing the Enemy and Qin Na

Application 1

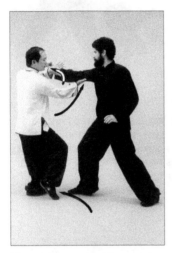 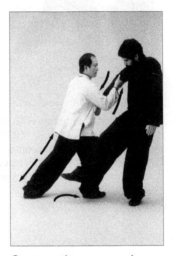

Your opponent strikes you with his right hand. Use your left forearm to deflect and lead it to the side, and at the same time place your right hand under his right elbow. Your right leg moves near your left leg to prevent your opponent from kicking your groin.

Once you have set up the correct position, immediately step forward, moving your left hand down and raising your right hand. Your opponent is now locked. Because his left hand is free, he will probably try to punch you. In this case, lift his arm to destroy his root and throw him away.

Application 2

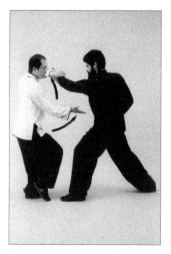 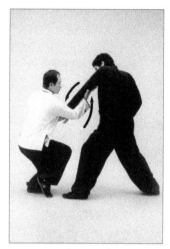

Your opponent punches with his left hand and steps forward with his left leg. Use your left forearm to deflect and lead it to the side, and at the same time place your right hand under his right elbow. Your right leg moves near your left leg to prevent your opponent from kicking your groin.

Cavity Strike or Striking the Vital Points

Application 1

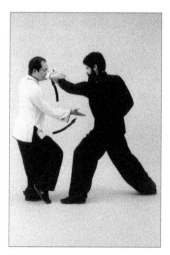 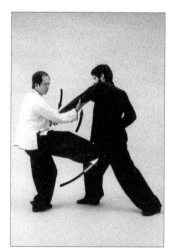

Your opponent punches with his left hand and steps forward with his left leg. Use your left forearm to deflect and lead it to the side, and at the same time place your right hand under his right elbow. After you lock your opponent's arm, your right leg can kick his groin or knee.

Application 2

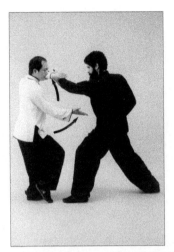 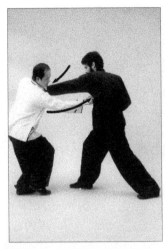

Your opponent punches with his left hand and steps forward with his left leg. Grasp and straighten your opponent's arm. His armpit or chest should be exposed to attack. Immediately after you deflect, use your right hand to strike while your left hand controls his wrist.

8. The Crane Spreads Its Wings (Bai He Liang Chi, 白鶴亮翅)

The Chinese name of this posture is bai he liang chi, which means white crane spreads wings. White cranes are very common in China and are well regarded by the people. When a crane fights, it usually blocks with its wings and attacks with both beak and wings. The wings derive their power from a shaking or jerking motion that starts in the body and passes to the wings. This is the same motion the crane uses to shake off water after it rains. The crane is not a muscular or strong bird, but when it strikes with its wings, it can break branches and kill or injure its enemy. In order to have this kind of strong jerking power, one must have an extremely strong root. Cranes have an inborn ability to maintain balance. They can often be seen perched on tree branches or bamboo. No matter how strong the wind blows and the branch shakes, the crane will remain there without falling.

Movements:

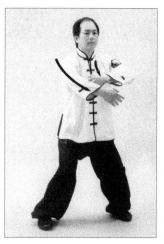

With both feet parallel, cross both arms in front of your chest.

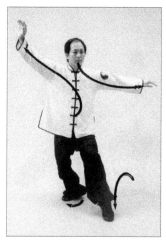

Rotate your right foot to the side and shift your weight to it, then step your left leg forward and touch the toes to the floor as both arms spread apart to the sides.

Analysis:

Moving your hands to your chest seals your chest area to protect it from attack. The strongest part of the crane's body is its wings; therefore, that is what it uses to block and to seal the opponent's attack. Once you have prevented the opponent from continuing his attack, you can then use your wings (hands and arms) to spread your opponent's attack to the sides. This will open the front of your opponent's body to attack.

Downing the Enemy

Application 1

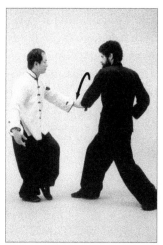

Your opponent attacks with his left hand. Deflect and grasp his left wrist with your left hand and pull it down.

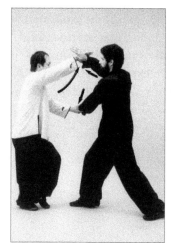

Now both your face and your opponent's face are exposed to attack. You can attack his eyes with your right hand to force him to block, or you can wait for his right hand to attack. In either case, control his right wrist.

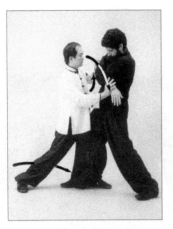 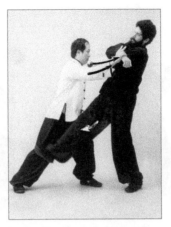

After you have set up this position, step your left leg behind the opponent's right leg, and at the same time move your right hand down and your left hand up to lock both of your opponent's hands.

Immediately push both your hands forward and upward and at the same time bounce your left thigh against his front leg to pull up his front root.

Qin Na Control

Application 1

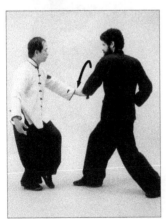 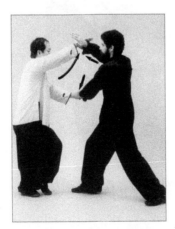 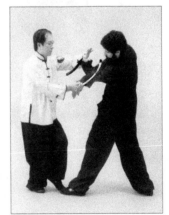

Your opponent attacks with his left hand. Deflect and grasp his left wrist with your left hand and pull it down. Control his right wrist.

After you have grabbed your opponent's wrists, rotate his right arm so that it stays straight and pull it down. As you do this, also raise your left hand to lock both his arms.

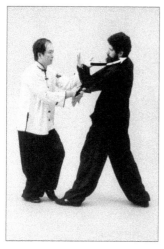 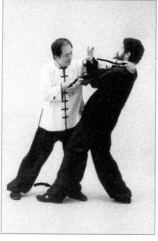 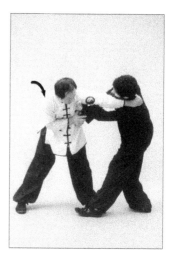

If you desire, you can continue your left hand movement to move it to the opponent's neck and use your upper left arm to control his left arm.

Finally, bend forward to completely lock him up.

Cavity Strike or Striking the Vital Points

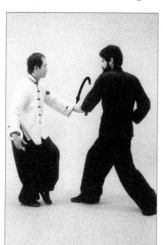 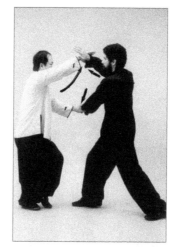 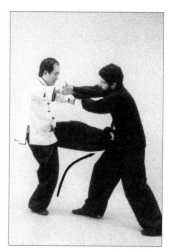

Deflect and grasp his left wrist with your left hand and pull it down. Control both wrists.

Use your left leg to kick his groin.

Technique 2

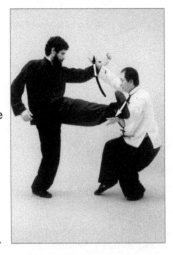

The spreading motion of crane spreads wings is commonly used to block double strikes. For example, it can be used to block a simultaneous punch and kick.

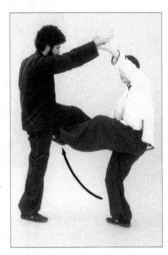

You can follow this by kicking him in the groin with your left leg.

9. Brush Knee and Step Forward (Lou Xi Yao Bu, 摟膝拗步)

The Chinese name of this form is lou xi yao bu. Lou in Chinese means to embrace, and xi means knee; therefore, lou xi means to embrace your knee. Yao means to twist or twist off, and is commonly used in expressions such as yao zhe (拗折) or yao duan (拗斷), which mean to break off by twisting. Bu means step; therefore, yao bu means to step forward with a twisting motion. The name of this form can therefore be better translated as "embrace knee and twist step."

Movements:

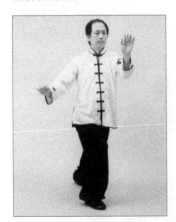
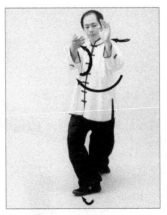

Beginning with your left hand and right foot forward, twist your body to the right and lift your right hand, while at the same time pushing your left hand slightly to the right.

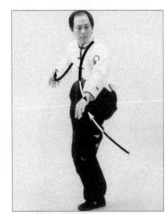

Raise your left leg while your left hand continues to circle down in front of the lifted knee.

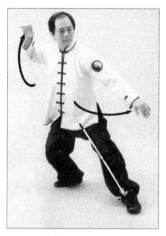 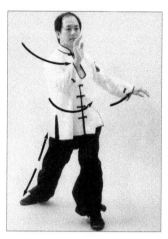

Your left hand continues on to your left side and your right hand circles up behind your ear while your left leg is stepping forward.

Finally, shift your weight forward and use your right hand to push forward.

Analysis:

When you are in the starting position of brush knee, your groin and right chest are open to attack. In order to seal these two places, pull your left knee up to seal the groin and twist your body to the right to hide your chest. Once you are in this position, your left leg is alive for kicking. Alternatively, step your left leg down behind your opponent's front leg to stop him from retreating, and at the same time use your right hand to strike.

Downing the Enemy

Application 1

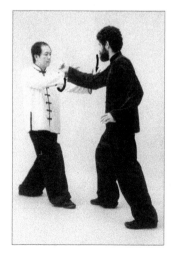

Your opponent punches your chest. Use your right hand to deflect and lead, and at the same time use your left hand to push his elbow to seal it and prevent further attack.

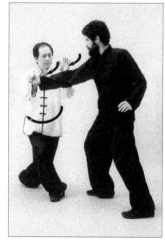

Twist your body to the right to lead his power past you.

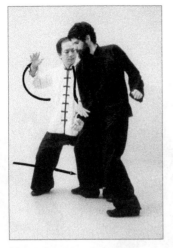 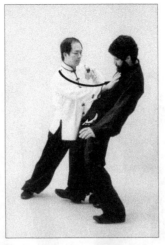

Next step your left leg behind his right leg while you push your left hand down to immobilize his right hand.

Finally, use your right hand to push his chest forward and downward while your left thigh bounces against his right leg to uproot his front leg.

Application 2

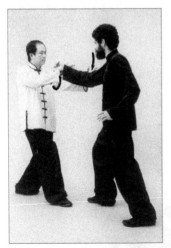 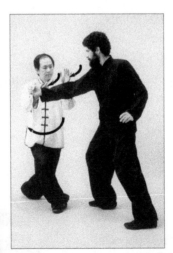 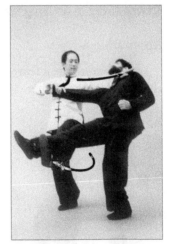

Neutralize the opponent's punch.

Use your left leg to sweep his right leg while your left hand moves to his neck and pushes downward.

Qin Na Control

Application 1

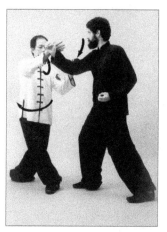 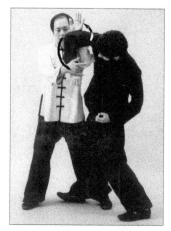 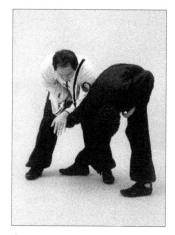

Your opponent punches toward your chest with his right hand. Neutralize his punch to the right.

Pull your right hand down and file your left hand up against his elbow, while your left leg steps to the inside of his right leg.

Continue twisting his arm and bow your body forward. If you wish to make him fall, sweep your left leg backward.

Cavity Strike or Striking the Vital Points

Application 1

In downing the enemy, application 1, instead of pushing downward, you may strike the solar plexus or other vital cavities on the chest.

Application 2

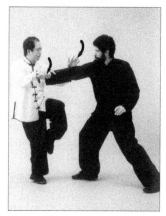 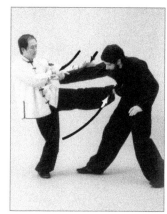

Your opponent punches toward your chest with his right hand. Neutralize his punch to the right. Grab his wrist.

You can then kick to break his front knee, or kick his stomach area to seal his breath.

Application 3

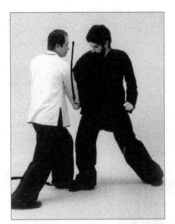 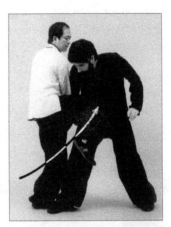

Alternatively, you can also use your knee to kick his stomach or chest areas.

10. Play the Guitar (Shou Hui Pi Pa, 手揮琵琶)

This form is called shou hui pi pa. Shou means hands, and hui means to strum on. The pi pa is a Chinese musical instrument, known as a balloon guitar. When the pi pa is played, it is held vertically in front of the chest, not against the abdomen like a Western guitar.

Movements:

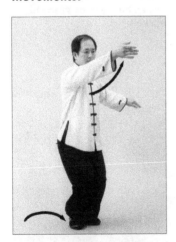 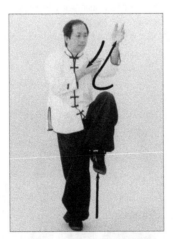 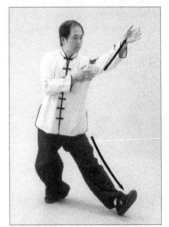

From the brush knee posture, step your right leg forward next to the left leg, and at the same time raise your right hand in front of your chest. Then move your left hand up and slide it forward under the right arm, while pulling your right hand into your chest. As you are moving your hands past each other, raise your left leg up. Finally, step your left leg forward and touch the floor with the heel, placing no weight on it.

Analysis:

When your opponent punches, first raise your right hand to lift up his punch and open his chest area to attack. Because both feet are together when you deflect, you can easily use either leg for kicking. Your left hand can either control his arm or strike.

Downing the Enemy

Application 1

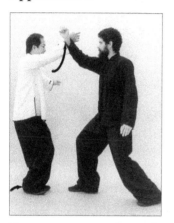
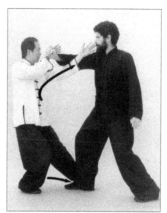
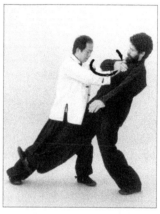

Your opponent punches with his right hand. Raise your right arm to neutralize his punch upward, and at the same time move your right leg forward to your left leg.

Immediately slide your left hand forward inside the opponent's elbow and at the same time place your left leg behind his right leg.

Then press your right hand forward against his chest, while your left hand either hooks his neck or grabs his upper arm.

Application 2

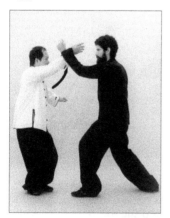
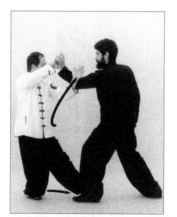
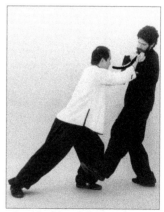

Your opponent punches you with his left hand with either his left leg or right leg forward. Deflect the punch and immediately slide your left hand forward. Next press your right hand forward.

Qin Na Control

Application 1

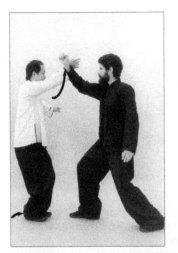 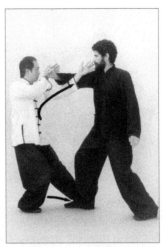

Your opponent punches with his right hand. Neutralize his punch upward and at the same time move your right leg forward to your left leg. Immediately slide your left hand forward inside the opponent's elbow and at the same time place your left leg behind his right leg.

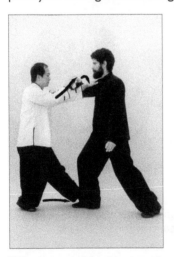 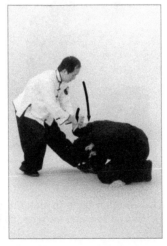

When your left hand moves into the opponent's elbow, grasp his right wrist with your right hand. Next push your left hand down and at the same time use your right hand to bend his right wrist until he is controlled.

Application 2

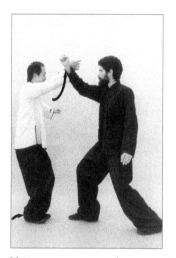 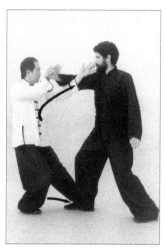

Your opponent punches you with his left hand with either his left leg or right leg forward. Deflect the punch, and immediately slide your left hand forward and at the same time place your left leg behind his right leg.

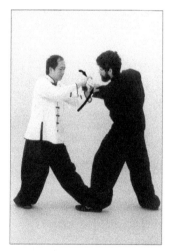 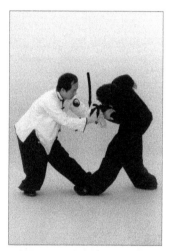

Use your left hand to lock the opponent's elbow and your right hand to bend his wrist to control him.

Cavity Strike or Striking the Vital Points

Application 1

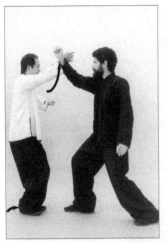 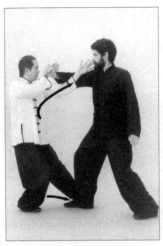 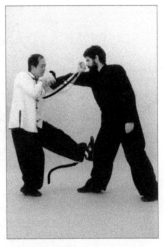

Raise your right arm to neutralize upward your opponent's punch and at the same time move your right leg forward to your left leg. Immediately slide your left hand forward and at the same time place your left leg behind his right leg.

Grab his right wrist with your right hand, and then strike his face with your left fist and break his knee with your left foot.

Application 2

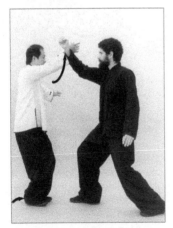 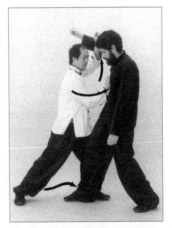

Raise your right arm to neutralize your opponent's punch upward and at the same time move your right leg forward to your left leg.

Step your left leg behind his right leg and move your left hand up to expose his chest for your right-hand strike.

Application 3

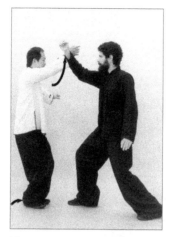

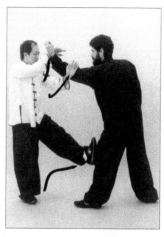

Your opponent punches you with his left hand. Neutralize the punch upward.

Next move your left hand in to lock his elbow and kick his knee with your left leg.

Application 4

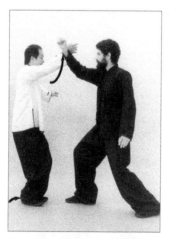

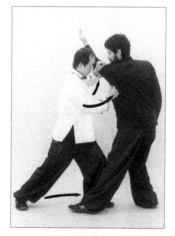

Your opponent punches you with his left hand. Neutralize upward.

Step your left leg forward and immediately punch under his armpit.

11. Twist Body and Circle Fist (Pie Shen Chui, 撇身捶)

This form is called pie shen chui. Pie means to twist or swing aside. It is commonly used in expressions such as pie kai (撇開), which means to set something aside or push it away. Shen means body, and chui means to strike. Therefore, this form should be translated as "twist your body and strike." This name tells you that in this form you must first turn your body to evade the opponent's attack, and then use your fist to strike the opponent's striking hand or even his body. This form is generally used together with the next form—step forward, deflect downward, parry, and punch—therefore, the applications of these two forms will be discussed together.

12. Step Forward, Deflect Downward, Parry, and Punch (Jin Bu Ban Lan Chui, 進步搬攔捶)

This form is called jin bu ban lan chui in Chinese. Jin bu means to move forward; ban means to remove or shift; lan means to hinder, obstruct, intercept, block, or cut off; and chui means to punch. The translation of this form should therefore be "step forward, remove, intercept, and punch." After doing the previous form, twist body and circle fist, in which you turn your body to evade the attack and punch your opponent from the side, or else push his punch to the side, the name of this form tells you to continue your movements by stepping forward, moving the opponent's punch to the side, hindering any further action, and punching him. From this explanation you can see that from the beginning, when your hand first touches your opponent's hand, you use a few techniques to lead his punch to the side, stick with him and hinder him, and finally strike him.

Movements:

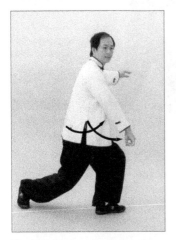

First twist your body to the left as you lower your right fist. This will move your body out of the way of the opponent's punch and lead it to the side.

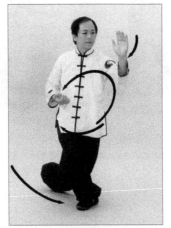

Your right hand continues to circle upward and then down to your waist while you step your right leg forward. Your left hand intercepts the opponent's attack by circling down to your right front.

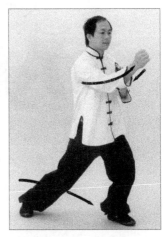

Your left leg then steps forward and your right hand punches past your left hand.

Analysis:

These forms are used to connect and then adhere and stick at close range. You first evade the opponent's attack by twisting your body to the side; your right arm moves out to seal your chest. After your opponent's punch has missed, he will immediately attempt to pull his hand back. In order to maintain the connection with your opponent, circle your right hand to your right and at the same time take two steps forward. This allows you to stick to your opponent's hand as he pulls it back, as well as lock his leg with your second step. Because your adhering and sticking have placed your opponent in a passive position, immediately use your left hand to push his arm down or to the side to allow your right hand to strike. This form is similar to brush knee and step forward, except that it is for short range while brush knee is for medium range.

Downing the Enemy

Application 1

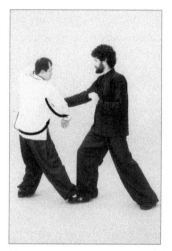 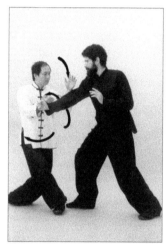

Your opponent punches with his right hand. Evade the punch by turning your body to the left.

Next twist your body to your right while circling your right hand clockwise to move his arm to your right.

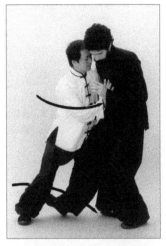 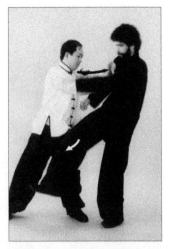

Immediately step your left leg behind his right leg while your left hand pushes down to open the opponent's chest, and your right hand moves to his chest.

Finally, push him forward and upward with your right hand as you bounce your left thigh against his right leg to uproot his right foot.

Qin Na Control

Application 1

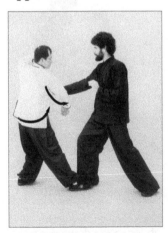 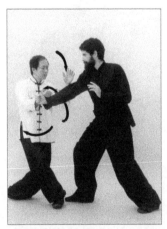 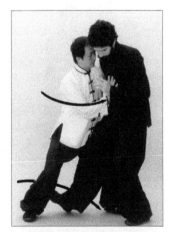

Your opponent punches with his right hand. Evade the punch by turning your body to the left.

Next twist your body to your right while circling your right hand clockwise to move his arm to your right.

Immediately step your left leg behind his right leg while your left hand pushes down to open the opponent's chest, and your right hand moves to his chest.

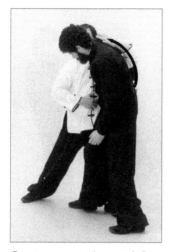

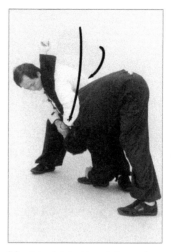

Continue to circle your left hand to the back of your opponent's right shoulder.

Next twist to the right and push your left hand down to control his right shoulder.

Cavity Strike or Striking the Vital Points

Application 1

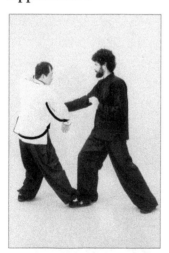

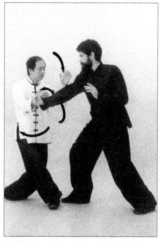

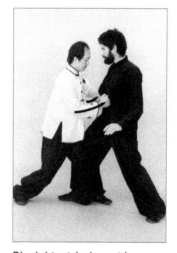

Your opponent punches with his right hand. Evade the punch by turning your body to the left.

Next twist your body to your right while circling your right hand clockwise to move his arm to your right.

Block his right leg with your left leg, press down with your left hand to control his arm and punch over it.

Application 2

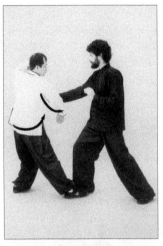

Your opponent punches with his right hand. Evade the punch by turning your body to the left.

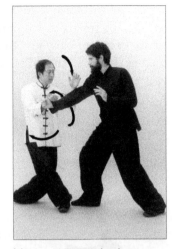

Next twist your body to your right while circling your right hand clockwise to move his arm to your right.

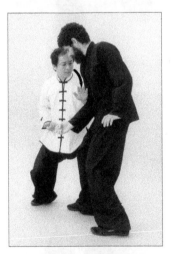

Step your left leg forward and your left hand pushes the opponent's right hand down.

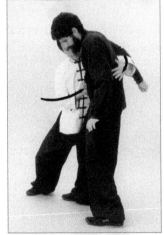

Continue to circle your left hand around to the opponent's back and use your right hand to punch his chest as your left hand pulls him forward.

13. Seal Tightly (Ru Feng Si Bi, 如封似閉)

The Chinese name of this form is ru feng si bi. Ru means like, if, or as. Feng means to seal up or blockade. Therefore, ru feng means "as if sealing up." Si in Chinese means like, as if, or seem to. Bi means close up. Therefore, si bi means "as if closing up." Therefore, the translation of this form should be "as if sealing, as if closing up."

Movements:

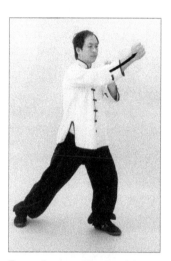 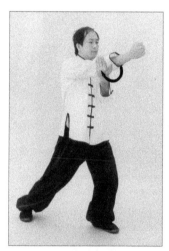

From the punching position, move your left hand to the outside of your right elbow.

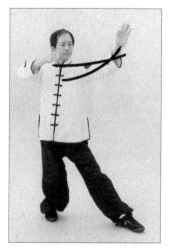 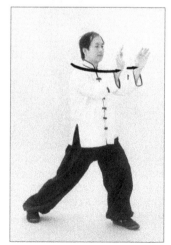

Next sit back and pull your right hand back as you turn your left palm forward and push it forward.

Finally, push your right hand forward.

Analysis:

This form is commonly used to nullify the opponent's grabbing, coiling, wrapping, or drilling.

Downing the Enemy

Application 1

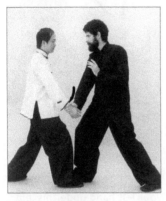

Your opponent grabs your right wrist.

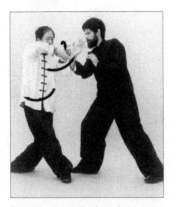

Raise your right hand to your chest and start rotating it in a counterclockwise direction. As you are doing this, twist your body to the right to prevent him from attacking you with his left hand, and place your left hand under his right hand.

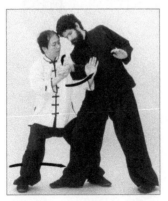

Continue rotating your right hand until you can grasp your opponent's wrist, and step your left leg behind his right leg.

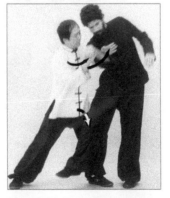

Finally, bounce the opponent away using your left wardoff and your right hand. Your left thigh should bounce against the opponent's right leg to help uproot it.

Application 2

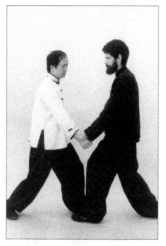

Your opponent grabs your right wrist with his left hand.

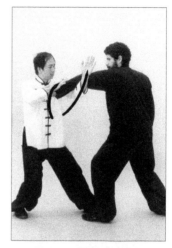

Rotate your right hand in a counterclockwise direction and at the same time place your left hand under his left elbow.

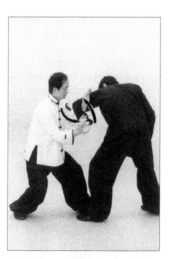

Continue rotating your right hand until you can grasp his left wrist, and then push it forward to bend his elbow.

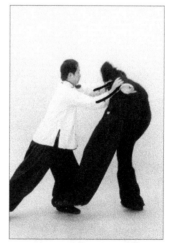

Finally, push forward with both hands to bounce him away.

14. Embrace Tiger and Return to the Mountain (Bao Hu Gui Shan, 抱虎歸山)

The Chinese name of this form is bao hu gui shan and means "embrace tiger and return to the mountain." The tiger is a very dangerous animal, and to say that you are embracing one implies that you are embracing an enemy. In order to embrace a tiger safely, you must hold him close and tight so that he cannot claw you. You must do the same thing when you embrace an opponent—you must hold him close so that he cannot hurt you. Return to the mountain implies that it is a long way to return home, and that this form is therefore a long jing. A short jing will not work. To return home with a tiger, you have to carry him, which tells you that this form is meant to destroy the opponent's root.

Movements:

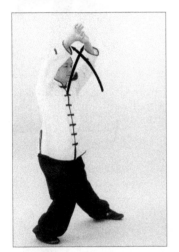 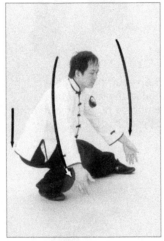 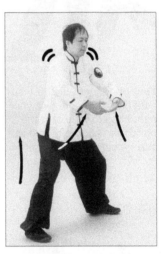

Raise your arms over your head and circle them down as you squat down on your right leg.

Finally, stand up while lifting both hands.

Downning the Enemy

Application 1

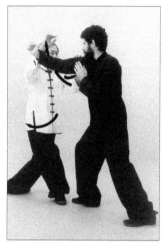 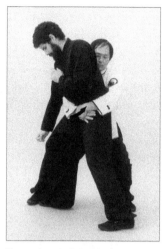 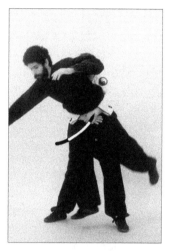

Your opponent punches you with his right hand. Use your right hand to intercept the punch and your left hand to seal his elbow or upper arm.

Step your left leg behind him and at the same time embrace his waist with both of your hands.

Finally, lift him up and, if you wish, throw him to the ground.

Application 2

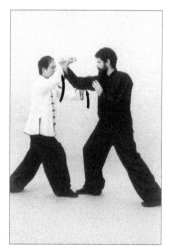 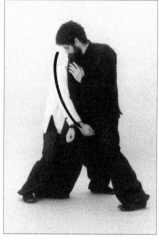 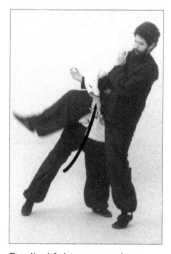

Deflect your opponent's punch.

Continue to press his right arm down. Step behind his right leg with your left leg and encircle his leg with both hands.

Finally, lift him up to destroy his root.

Qin Na Control

Application 1

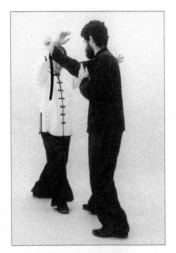

Deflect the opponent's punch.

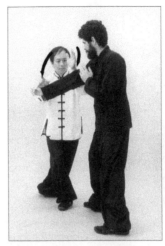

Press his arm down with your left hand.

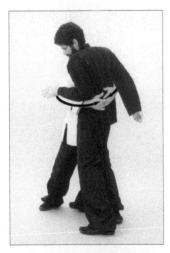

As you step behind his right leg with your left leg, continue to circle your hands around him and place both hands on his lower back.

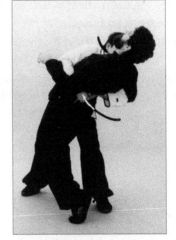

Pull both hands in toward your stomach while bending your body forward and pressing his chest with your chin.

Cavity Strike or Striking the Vital Points

Application 1

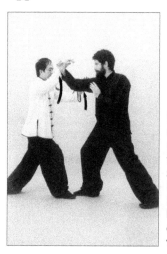

Deflect your opponent's punch. Continue to press his right arm down. Step behind his right leg with your left leg and encircle his leg with both hands.

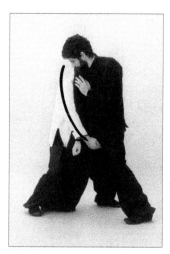

When you are on your opponent's side, you can strike his groin.

Transition Form between the Parts (Guo Du Shi, 過渡勢)

In Yang-style taijiquan there is no name for this transition. It is very similar to the form white snake turns body and spits poison, which is in part three of the sequence (form 32 in this chapter); however, there are two differences. First, in the beginning of this form, only the toes of the right foot touch the floor, and there is no weight on the foot, whereas in the form white snake turns, both feet are flat on the floor. Second, the jing that is applied in this form is a long jing, while white snake turns uses short, fast jing.

Movements:

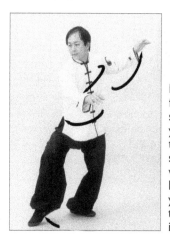

From a forward-facing stance, turn your body to the right while shifting your weight to the left foot so that your right toes touch the floor in a false stance.

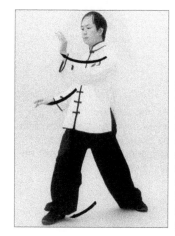

Step forward with your right leg into a mountain-climbing stance, deflect to the side with your right hand and push forward with your left hand.

Analysis:

Your root must be solid so that you can twist your body and generate jing. This will enable you to loosen up an opponent's bear hug or deflect an attack to the side. Once you have done this, you will have enough time to shift your root to the left, allowing your right foot to be alive for other applications.

Downing the Enemy

Application 1

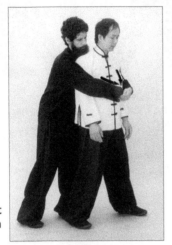

Your opponent grabs you from behind.

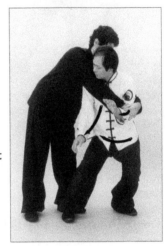

Squat down to build your root and generate jerking power. This will also loosen up the opponent's hold.

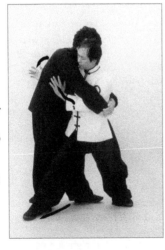

Next shift your weight to the left and step to the outside of his right leg with your right leg, and hold his body with both your hands.

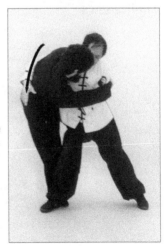

Once you have set up this position, generate power from your legs and waist and twist him over your leg.

Qin Na Control

Application 1

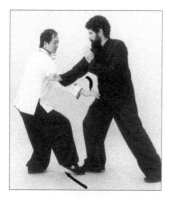 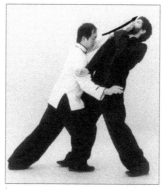 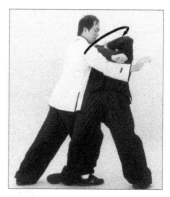

Your opponent strikes your waist from the side or rear. Twist your body and sit back on the rear foot, and at the same time brush his punch away. The toes of your right foot should be lightly touching the floor.

Attack his face with your left hand and block his right leg with your right leg.

Next use your left arm to circle his neck and press down.

Cavity Strike or Striking the Vital Points

Application 1

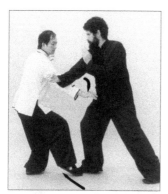 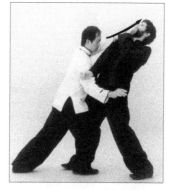

Deflect your opponent's punch to your waist. Sit back on your rear leg into a false stance.

You now have several options for your counterattack. For example, your right leg can kick his knee or groin, or else you can block his right leg with your right leg and strike his face. Alternatively, your right hand can also attack his groin.

15. Punch under the Elbow (Zhou Di Kan Chui, 肘底看捶)

The Chinese name of this form is zhou di kan chui. Zhou is elbow, di is bottom, kan is look, and chui is punch or strike. The name therefore means "look at the punch under the elbow" and implies "beware of the punch from under the elbow."

Movements:

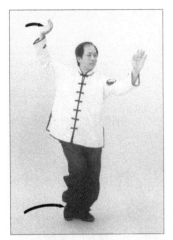 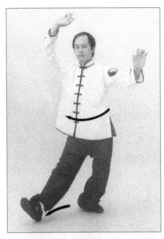 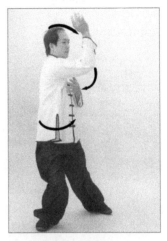

From the end of the single whip posture, move your right leg up to the left leg, while your left hand is in front of your chest and your right hand rises above your head.

Turn right and step your right leg forward.

Immediately shift your weight to the right leg and twist your body to the left, and at the same time move your right hand down across your face while your left hand moves to the front of your chest.

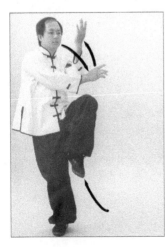 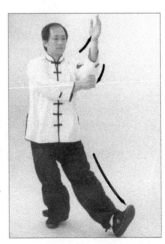

Continue the movement by pressing your right hand down and lifting your left hand up and out, while at the same time you raise your left leg.

Finally, place your right hand underneath your left elbow and form a taijiquan fist, and lower your left leg to the floor, touching with the heel.

Analysis:

The first step in this form is a yielding movement. Avoid the opponent's attack by stepping to the side, while using your hands to neutralize the opponent's attack and trap his hands. Your left hand can attack the opponent's face and your right hand can strike his chest. Your left leg has no weight on it and can be used for kicking.

Downing the Enemy

Application 1

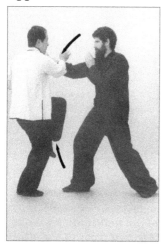 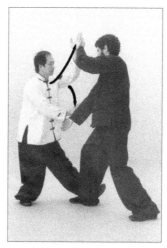 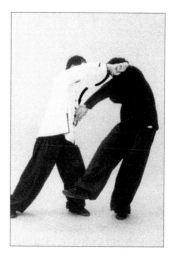

Your opponent punches with his right hand. Use your right hand to press it down while moving your left leg up.

Next use your left hand to slap his face, and at the same time seal his right leg with your left leg to prevent his retreat. Your attack to his face forces your opponent to use his left hand to block.

Immediately grab his left wrist with your left hand and his right wrist with your right hand, and twist both his arms. Finally, push forward with both of your hands to bounce him away.

Qin Na Control

Application 1

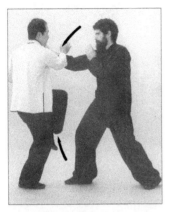 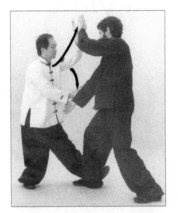 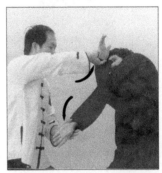

Your opponent punches with his right hand. Use your right hand to press it down while moving your left leg up.

Next use your left hand to slap his face, and at the same time seal his right leg with your left leg to prevent his retreat. Your attack to his face forces your opponent to use his left hand to block.

Cross the opponent's arms. Twist his left arm over his right arm to lock both arms.

Cavity Strike or Striking the Vital Points

Application 1

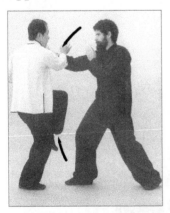 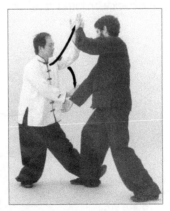 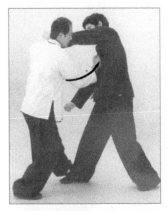

Your opponent punches with his right hand. Use your right hand to press it down while moving your left leg up.

Next use your left hand to slap his face, and at the same time seal his right leg with your left leg to prevent his retreat. Your attack to his face forces your opponent to use his left hand to block.

This exposes his chest, which you can strike with your right fist.

Application 2

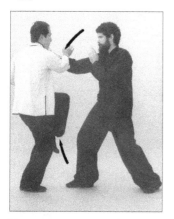

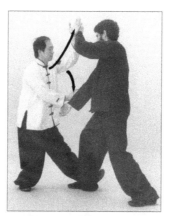

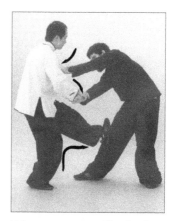

Your opponent punches with his right hand. Use your right hand to press it down while moving your left leg up.

Next use your left hand to slap his face, and at the same time seal his right leg with your left leg to prevent his retreat. Your attack to his face forces your opponent to use his left hand to block.

When you control both of the opponent's hands, you can use your left leg to break his knee.

16. Step Back and Repulse Monkey (Dao Nian Hou, 倒摔猴)

The Chinese name of this form is dao nian hou. Dao means to move backward, nian means to repel or drive away, and hou is monkey. Monkeys specialize in grabbing and sticking. The name of this form tells you that it is used when someone is trying to grab your hands or arms and you move backward and fend him off.

Movements:

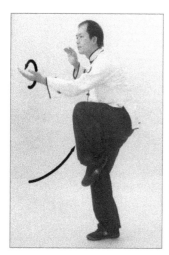

When your left hand and leg are forward, first rotate your left hand so that the palm faces up while raising your left leg and preparing to withdraw.

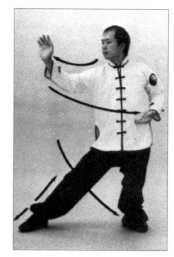

Touch your left leg down behind you and sit back into a four-six stance, and at the same time pull your left hand back to your waist while your right hand pushes forward.

Analysis:

The first motion of this form is to twist your hand out of the opponent's grasp and to grasp his arm. Raising your leg prepares you for either kicking or retreating. Once you have stepped back, you can control the opponent's arm and either strike him or knock him down.

Downing the Enemy

Application 1

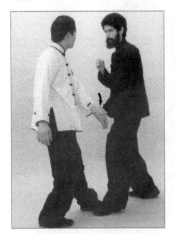 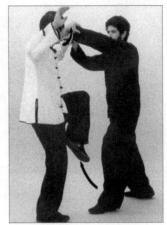 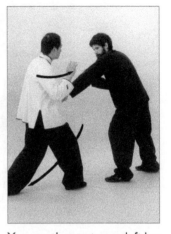

Your opponent grabs your left wrist with his left hand and prepares to punch you with his right fist.

Immediately raise your left hand and rotate the palm up to escape from his grab, and then grasp his wrist while lifting your left leg. This automatically blocks his punch and exposes his stomach to your kick.

You can then put your left leg down behind you and sit back while pulling your left hand back to your waist.

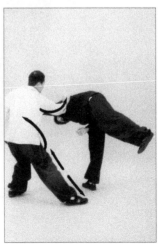

This will pull your opponent off balance. In order to prevent him from attacking with his elbow or shoulder, place your right hand by his armpit and twist your body to the left to make him fall.

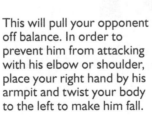

Qin Na Control

Application 1

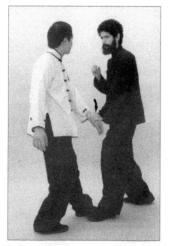

Your opponent grabs your left wrist with his left hand and prepares to punch you with his right fist.

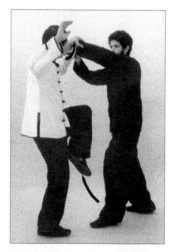

Immediately raise your left hand and rotate the palm up to escape from his grab, and then grasp his wrist for control while lifting your left leg.

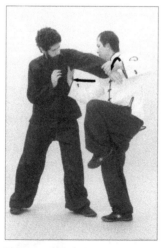

Place your right hand in the area of his armpit.

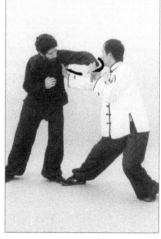

Then sit back and use your left hand to bend his left wrist to control him.

Cavity Strike or Striking the Vital Points

Application 1

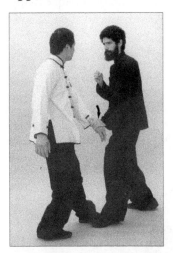 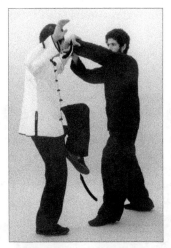 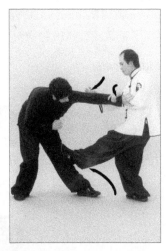

Your opponent grabs your left wrist with his left hand and prepares to punch you with his right fist.

Immediately raise your left hand and rotate the palm up to escape from his grab, and then grasp his wrist for control while lifting your left leg.

After you have grabbed the opponent's wrist with your left hand, use your left leg to kick his stomach or knee.

Application 2

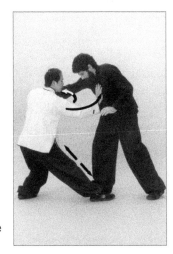

If your opponent grabs your left hand with his right hand, you can rotate your left palm up to open his chest and immediately sit back and strike his chest with your right palm.

17. Diagonal Flying (Xie Fei Shi, 斜飛勢)

The Chinese name of this form is xie fei shi. Xie means slanted, inclined, or oblique; fei means to fly; and shi means posture. Therefore, the translation should be "oblique flying posture." The name tells you that when you use this posture your arms move out diagonally as if you were flying.

Movements:

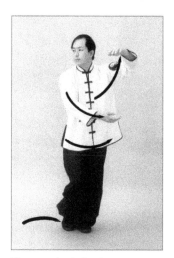 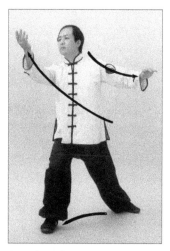

Turn to the left, drawing your right arm and leg back, and raising your left arm.

Step forward with your right leg. As you shift forward, turn your body to the right, raise your right arm, and lower your left arm.

Analysis:

This form neutralizes an attack by deflecting with your left hand and twisting your body to the side. Your arm or shoulder is then used to push or bounce the opponent diagonally upward to uproot him and make him fall. When you defend, there is no weight on your right leg, so you can easily use it for kicking.

Downing the Enemy

Application 1

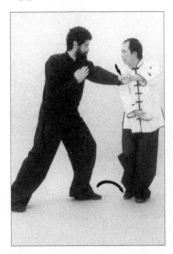 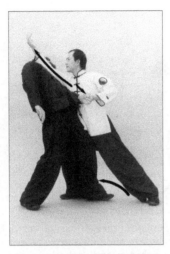 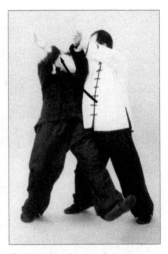

Your opponent punches you with his left hand. Use your left hand to intercept, grab, and pull it down.

Next step behind his left leg with your right leg, and at the same time slip your right arm above his left arm to press diagonally upward against his chest and neck.

If you intend to make your opponent fall, you should also use your right thigh to bounce and uproot his left leg.

Qin Na Control

Application 1

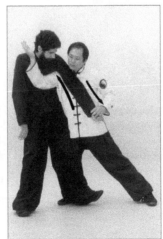

In the Downing the Enemy application, after your left hand has grasped his left wrist and pulled down, step behind his left leg with your right leg and at the same time push up with your shoulder to lock his shoulder. In order to make this application effective, your left hand must rotate the opponent's left arm until his palm faces up.

Cavity Strike or Striking the Vital Points

Application 1

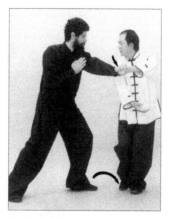 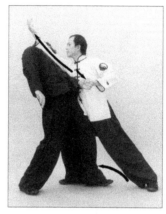

Your opponent punches you with his left hand. Use your left hand to intercept, grab, and pull it down. Next step behind his left leg with your right leg, and at the same time slip your right arm above his left arm to press diagonally upward against his chest and neck.

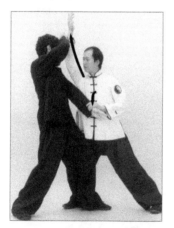 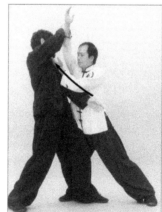

If he uses his right hand to stop your attempt, use your left hand to stab his throat or file his neck.

18. Pick Up Needle from Sea Bottom (Hai Di Lao Zhen, 海底撈針)

The Chinese name of this form is hai di lao zhen. Hai di means sea bottom, lao means to scoop up, and zhen means needle. Therefore, the translation of this form is "scoop up needle from the sea bottom." According to Chinese custom, the top of the head is called tian ling gai (天靈蓋) and means heaven spirit cover. The perineum is called hai di (海底)

and means sea bottom. Therefore, the name of this form indicates that you are attacking the groin from below.

Movements:

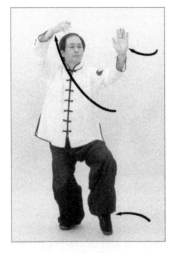

Sit back onto your right leg into a false stance and at the same time raise both hands.

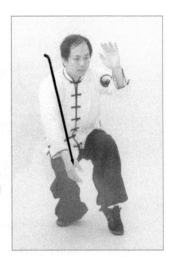

Next lower your body and drop your right hand down to knee level.

Analysis:

When your opponent attacks high, pull back your body and use both hands to intercept and deflect his attack. His right side is now exposed to attack. Because your left leg has no weight on it, it can be used for a quick kick. The dropping motion in this technique can also be used as a downward pluck.

Downing the Enemy

Application 1

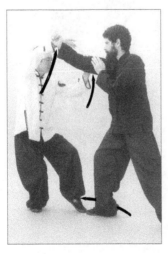

Draw back as your opponent punches you with his right hand. Intercept his attack with your right hand and press his elbow with your left hand.

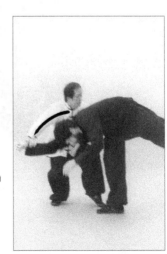

Grasp his arm by the wrist and elbow and pull him downward and past you.

Qin Na Control

Application 1

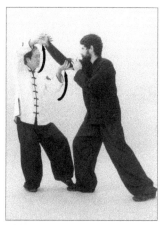 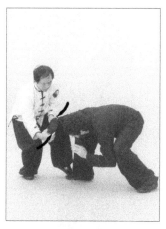

When your opponent strikes you with his right hand, intercept the punch with your right hand and press the elbow upward with your left hand.

Next bend his wrist with your right hand and squeeze his hand and elbow together as you push him down.

Cavity Strike or Striking the Vital Points

Application 1

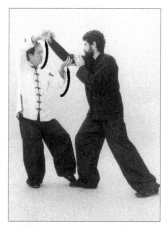 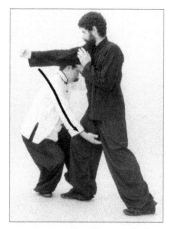

Deflect your opponent's strike upward.

Grab his groin with your right hand and pull it upward.

Application 2

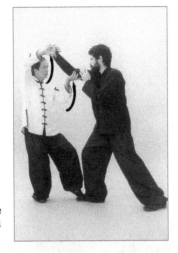

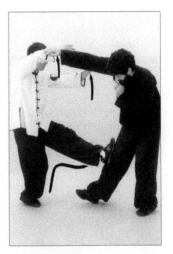

Deflect the opponent's attack.

Use your left leg to kick his knee.

19. Fan Back (Shan Tong Bei, 扇通背)

The Chinese name of this form is shan tong bei. Shan means fan, tong means through or reachable, and bei means back. In China there is a kind of monkey with very long arms. Their arms are so long that they can easily scratch their backs, and so they are called tong bei yuan (通背猿), which means reach-the-back apes, or tong bi yuan (通臂猿), which means reachable-arm apes. This indicates that when you use this form, your arms are long and stretched out far, and therefore the jing is a long jing. When you draw back in the first part of this form, you should arc your back to accumulate as much jing as possible, then when you straighten out, you extend your arms like a Chinese fan.

Movements:

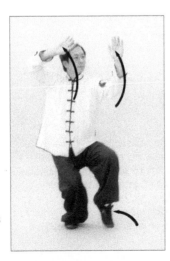

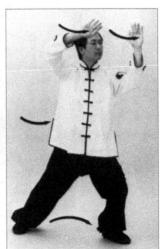

Draw your body back, with only the toes of the left foot touching the floor, and use both hands to intercept and deflect.

Immediately step your left leg forward and at the same time push both of your hands forward.

Analysis:

This form is generally used for close range. After you neutralize the opponent's attack, use both hands to push him off balance.

Downing the Enemy

Application 1

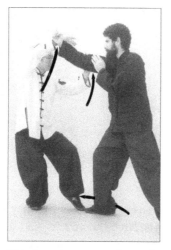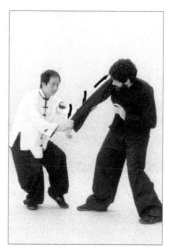

This form is commonly used together with the previous form, pick up needle from sea bottom. Draw back as your opponent punches you with his right hand. Intercept his attack with your right hand and press his elbow with your left hand. Pull the opponent's right arm downward.

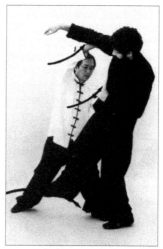

If he resists and pulls back, follow his pull and use both hands to push him off balance. If the fighting range is very close, you may also be able to block his right leg with your left leg to prevent his retreat.

Qin Na Control

Application 1

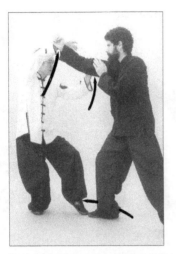 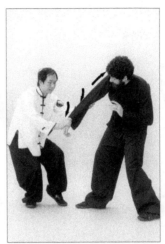

Draw back as your opponent punches you with his right hand. Intercept his attack with your right hand and press his elbow with your left hand. Pull the opponent's right arm downward.

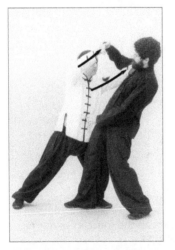 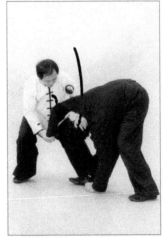

If he resists and pulls back, follow his pull and place your left hand on the back of the opponent's neck.

Press him down while bending his hand toward his elbow.

Cavity Strike or Striking the Vital Points

Application 1

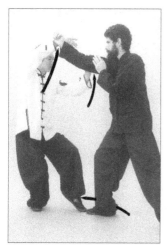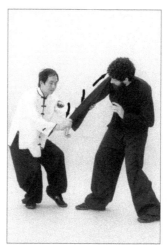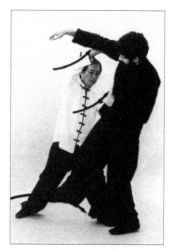

Draw back as your opponent punches you with his right hand. Intercept his attack with your right hand and press his elbow with your left hand. Pull the opponent's right arm downward. If he resists and pulls back, follow his pull.

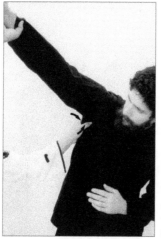

You can use your left hand to strike his throat or armpit, or to grab the muscles under his armpit.

20. Wave Hands in the Clouds (Yun Shou, 雲手)

The Chinese name of this form is yun shou and means cloud hands, which implies waving your hands like floating clouds. The movement of clouds can be fast or slow, but it is steady and continuous. Therefore, when you perform this form, you wave your hands the way clouds move. It is a long-range, continuous-jing application.

Movements:

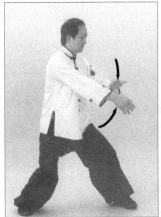
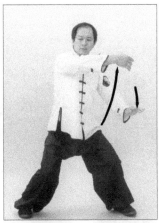
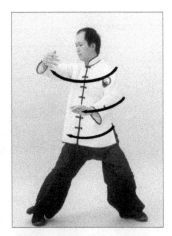

Stand in a horse stance and move your left hand down while raising your right hand up to your chest, palm facing inward.

Keeping your body central and upright, turn to the right while your hands maintain the same positional relationship to your body.

Analysis:

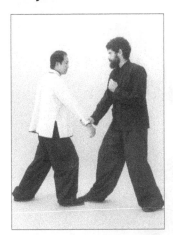
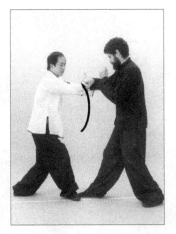
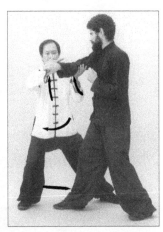

This form is designed for neutralizing the opponent's grabbing. Neutralize his grabbing to the side and also use your twisting jing to make him lose his balance. When you twist your body, it must be centered and balanced. For example, when your opponent grasps your right wrist with his right hand, raise your right hand up to your chest while your left hand presses on his elbow to prevent his using elbow stroke. You can step forward with your left leg or backward with your right leg while you are twisting your body.

Downing the Enemy

Application 1

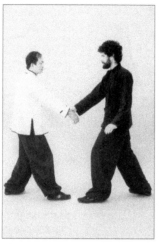

Your opponent grabs your right wrist with his right hand while his left leg is stepping forward.

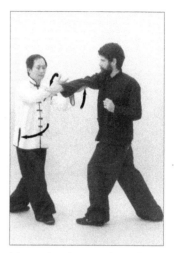

Neutralize him to the right.

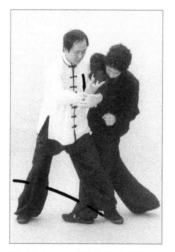

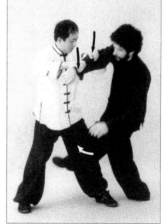

Next step behind his left leg with your left leg and immediately pull him down while bouncing your left thigh backward to uproot his left foot.

Qin Na Control

Application 1

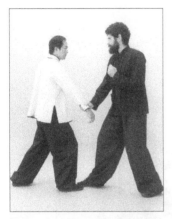 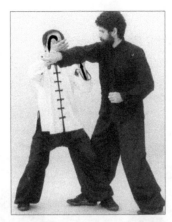 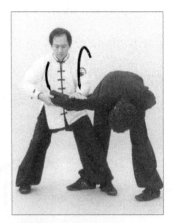

Your opponent grabs your right wrist with his right hand, right leg forward.

After you neutralize the grab, step in front of his right leg with your left leg.

Grasp his right wrist and press down on his elbow with your left hand. In this application, if you bounce or slide your left thigh backward, you can also make him fall.

21. Stand High to Search Out the Horse (Gao Tan Ma, 高探馬)

The Chinese name of this form is gao tan ma. Gao means high, tan means to try or search out, and ma means horse. When you search for your horse in the field, you must use your hands to shade your eyes from the sun in order to see far and clear. This indicates that the hands are used for blocking. The horse fights mainly by kicking, so the name implies that your leg can be used for kicking, and also that when you stand up high, your lower body is exposed to a kicking attack.

Movements:

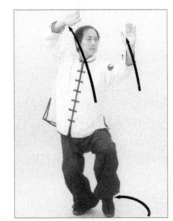

Sit back into the false stance as you draw your arms back and up.

Analysis:

This form is similar to the beginning of both pick up needle from sea bottom and fan back. The difference is that this form is applied in a shorter and quicker manner to set your opponent up for your kick.

Cavity Strike or Striking the Vital Points

Application 1

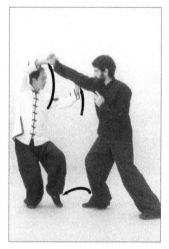

Your opponent punches you with his right hand. Use your right hand to slide the attack up and your left hand to push his elbow up, while you withdraw your left leg.

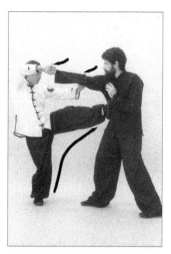

Immediately kick with your left leg to his knee or chest.

22. Separate Foot (Fen Jiao, 分腳)

The Chinese name of this form is fen jiao and means separate foot. It implies that the feet are separated sideward.

Movements:

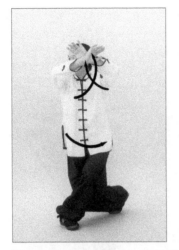 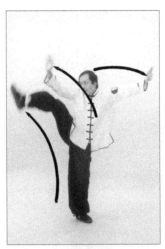

Twist your body to the side and scoop upward with both hands, and then kick out sideways.

Analysis:

In this form you must first deflect upward to protect yourself and to expose your opponent's side. If possible, grab your opponent's hand to prevent him from escaping or blocking.

Cavity Strike or Striking the Vital Points

Application 1

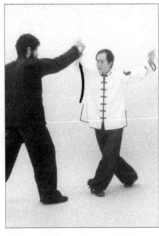 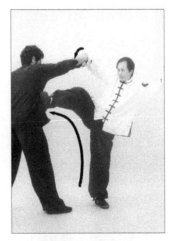

Your opponent punches with his right hand. Deflect up with your right hand and twist your body to the side.

Next grasp his wrist with your right hand and kick his side with your right leg.

23. Kick with Heel (Deng Jiao, 蹬腳)

The Chinese name of this form is deng jiao and means to use your heel to step or kick, usually forward.

Movements:

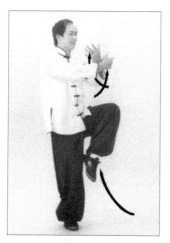
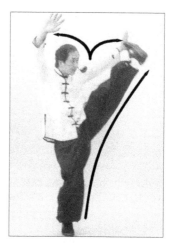

First cross your hands in front of your chest as you lift your left knee up. Next open both hands and kick forward with your heel.

Analysis:

Before you kick, you must seal all of your vital points from your opponent's strike. Therefore, first cross your hands in front of your chest to protect your chest area, and at the same time lift your left leg to protect your groin and dan tian. Then, if you have a suitable target, kick.

Cavity Strike or Striking the Vital Points

Application 1

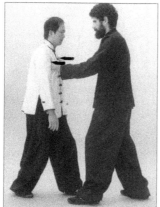

Your opponent grabs your shirt.

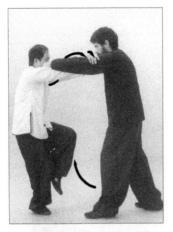 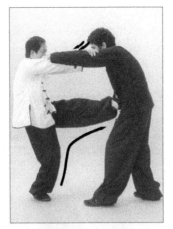

Deflect up and grab both his arms and at the same time raise your left leg.

Next immediately kick his groin or dan tian area. You must kick as soon and as fast as you can, because your opponent can also kick you.

24. Step Forward and Strike Down with the Fist (Jin Bu Zai Chui, 進步栽捶)

The Chinese name of this form is jin bu zai chui. Jin bu means to step forward, zai means to fall, and chui means to punch. There are not too many vital points in the lower body to strike. Common targets are the dan tian, groin, and upper thigh.

Movements:

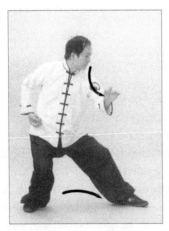 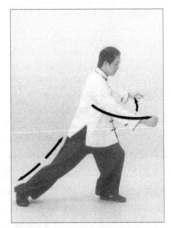

Step your left leg forward and use your left hand to brush sideward.

Once your hand is past your body, shift your body forward and strike downward with your fist.

Analysis:

This form is for deflecting low punches and kicks. After you deflect, shift your body forward close to your opponent to immobilize him. This will give you a good opportunity to strike.

Cavity Strike or Striking the Vital Points

Application 1

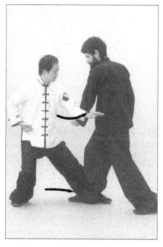

Your opponent punches with his left hand while his right leg is forward. Use your left hand to deflect it to the side and at the same time step your left leg behind his right leg.

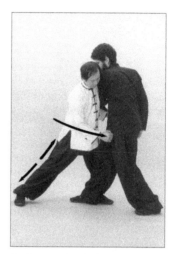

Shift your body forward and punch down to his groin.

25. Strike the Tiger (Da Hu, 打虎)

This form is called da hu in Chinese and means strike the tiger. The name of this form comes from the squatting stance called tame the tiger stance (fu hu bu, 伏虎步), which was popularized by Wu Song (武松), a famous fictional hero from the Song dynasty (宋朝) (960–1278 CE). One day Wu Song was walking down a path when he saw a sign on a tree warning of a tiger in the area, and urging people not to travel through the area alone. Wu Song, who was drunk at the time, looked at the sign and laughed. He thought it was only a trick to scare people into staying at a local hotel, so he ignored the sign and walked ahead. After a mile or so, a big tiger suddenly jumped out of the bushes right in front of him. Instantly, all the alcohol he had drunk became sweat, and he was totally awake. The only weapon he had to defend himself with was a short dagger. When the tiger leaped toward his face, he suddenly squatted down out of the way, and as the tiger passed over him, he stabbed his dagger into the tiger's stomach and killed it. Since then, this squatting stance has been called tame the tiger stance.

Movements:

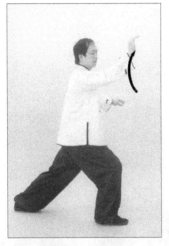

First deflect up with your right hand, palm out.

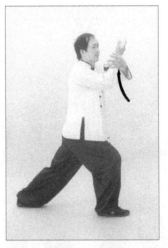

Next brush up the outside of the right arm with your left hand.

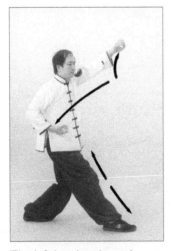

The left hand grabs and continues up, while your right hand pulls back to your waist and your body shifts back.

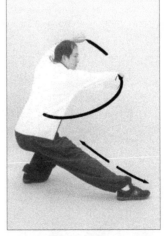

Finally, twist your body to the left and sink down on the left leg into the tame the tiger stance and strike with your right fist.

Analysis:

Your right hand deflects the attack and your left hand immediately takes over to put your opponent in a passive situation. Once you have the opportunity, pull him down to make him lose balance and use the other hand to strike him. Your root and your waist twisting jing are extremely important in this application.

Cavity Strike or Striking the Vital Points

Application 1

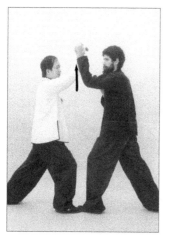 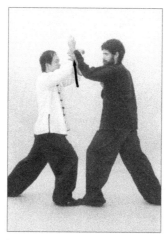 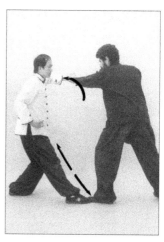

Your opponent punches with his left hand. Use your right hand to deflect upward.

Immediately pick up his momentum with your left hand.

Grab his left wrist and pull.

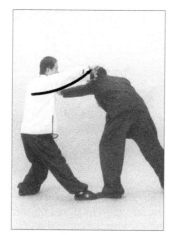 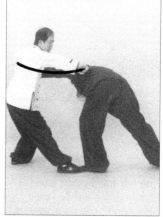

Once the opponent is exposed, twist your body to the left and strike with your right hand to his head or under the armpit.

26. Attack the Ears with the Fists (Shuang Feng Guan Er, 雙風貫耳)

The Chinese name of this form is shuang feng guan er. Shuang means a pair, double, or both; feng means the wind; guan means to go through or pass through; and er means ears. Therefore, the translation of this form should be "two winds pass through the ears." In this form, the fists generate the wind. The strikes must be fast and powerful to approach the targets, which are the temples or other cavities.

Movements:

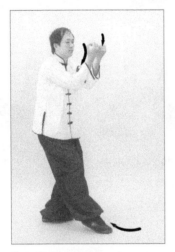

First bring both hands together in front of your chest as you sit back into a false stance.

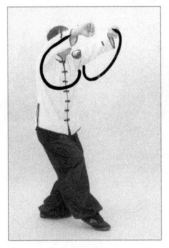

Then open your arms, make two fists, and strike the target with two circular strikes.

Analysis:

Bringing both hands in front of your chest seals it from your opponent's attack, and emptying your right leg gives you the opportunity to kick. Once you have sealed your opponent's strike, you can follow his striking limbs to attack his body or head.

Cavity Strike or Striking the Vital Points

Application 1

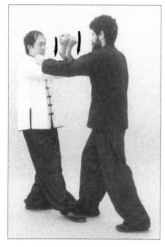 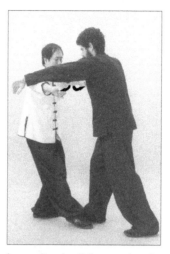 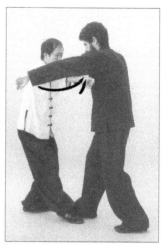

When your opponent strikes with both hands, deflect the strikes with both your arms.

Immediately slide your hands downward.

Strike him under the armpits.

Application 2

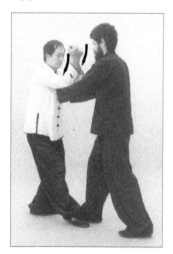 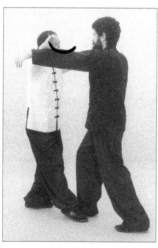 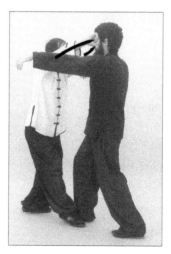

Your opponent grasps your shirt with both hands. Press his arms down with your elbows.

Next lead his hands to the sides.

Finally, strike his temples with both fists.

Application 3

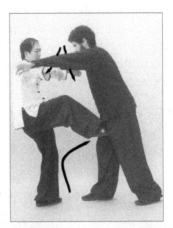

In the first and second applications, you can also easily use your right foot to kick his groin.

27. Wild Horses Shear the Mane (Ye Ma Fen Zong, 野馬分鬃)

The Chinese name of this form is ye ma fen zong. Ye means wild, ma means horse, fen means to shear or divide, and zong means mane. The horse is a powerful animal, and a wild horse is particularly forceful and vigorous. The name of this form gives the image of a horse tossing his head vigorously and shaking his mane. The word "shear" is used because when you do this form, you "tear" your hands apart as you turn your body. The motion is continuous, extended, and powerful. It is a long jing that can rend the opponent off his feet.

Movements:

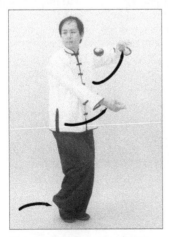

Turn to the left while raising your left hand and drawing your right foot back. The hands should be facing each other as if holding a basketball.

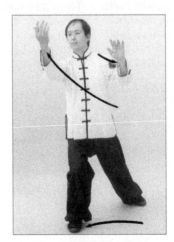

Step forward with your right foot and extend your right hand while drawing back your left hand.

Analysis:

In order to shear or divide your opponent, you must grasp part of his body, usually an arm, and pull it in one direction, and at the same time use your other arm against his body to move him in the other direction. Also, your right leg should be placed so that it blocks the opponent from retreating or kicking. This is an example of rend jing, because you move the opponent in two directions at once.

Downing the Enemy

Application 1

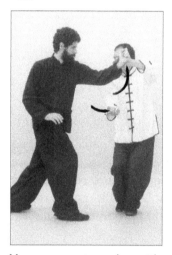 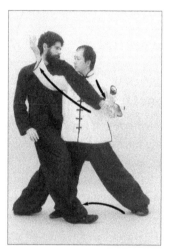 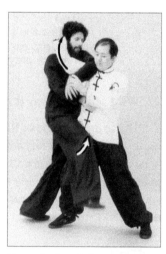

Your opponent punches with his left hand while his right leg steps forward. Intercept his attack and lead it to the left with your left hand while drawing your right leg in to protect yourself from a possible left kick.

Next step your right leg forward to the inside of his right leg and at the same time raise your right arm under his armpit.

To make him fall, rotate your body to the right while pushing his right knee to the left with your right knee.

Qin Na Control

Application 1

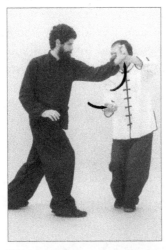 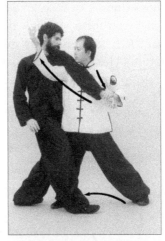

Your opponent punches with his left hand while his right leg steps forward. Intercept his attack and lead it to the left with your left hand while drawing your right leg in to protect yourself from a possible left kick.

Next step your right leg forward to the inside of his right leg and at the same time raise your right arm under his armpit. When you have your arm under your opponent's armpit, pull down with your left hand while raising your right shoulder.

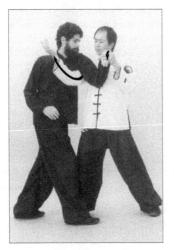 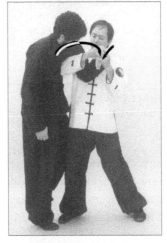

You can also bend his left elbow and wrist.

Immediately use both hands to bend his wrist.

28. Fair Lady Weaves with Shuttle (Yu Nu Chuan Suo, 玉女穿梭)

The Chinese name of this form is yu nu chuan suo. Yu is jade, and nu is girl or lady; together they refer to a fair or beautiful lady. Chuan means to thread or pass through, and suo is a weaver's shuttle. In order to weave a piece of cloth, you must move the horizontal threads back and forth through the vertical threads with a shuttle. As you do the repetitions of the form, your body moves back and forth as if you are working a loom. You have to watch carefully in order to insert the shuttle accurately through the threads.

Movements:

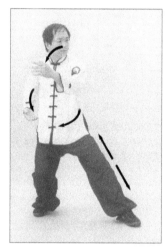 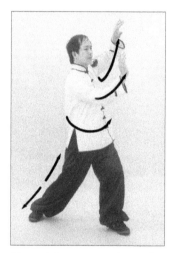

First shift your weight to your rear foot, sitting in a four-six stance, and at the same time turn your body to the right so that your left hand begins to move up in front of your chest and your right hand draws back to your waist.

Next shift your weight to the front foot and turn your body to the left, raising your left hand in front of your face and pushing your right hand to your left front.

Analysis:

This form is usually used at close range. From the movements of the form, it is understood that you are attacking the vital cavity in the armpit, where a correct strike can cause a heart attack. You must first expose the target by raising his elbow, and then use the secret sword hand form in order to reach the cavity, which is deep in the armpit.

Cavity Strike or Striking the Vital Points

Application 1

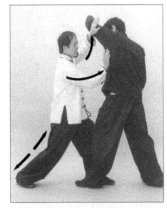

Your opponent punches or has his elbow raised. Use your forward hand to raise his elbow and simultaneously strike him with your rear hand.

29. Lower the Snake Body (She Shen Xia Shi, 蛇身下势)

The Chinese name of this form is she shen xia shi. She means snake, shen means body, xia means down or to lower, and shi means aspect or manner. The image is that of a snake wrapped around a branch, lowering its head as if about to attack. Therefore, the translation should be "snake creeps down." The name implies that you must first wrap, coil, stick, and adhere with your opponent before you lower your body to attack. When a snake creeps down a branch, its head is lower than its body, searching the air to find and attack its target. This means that you coil and wrap on the top while you attack your opponent's lower body.

Movements:

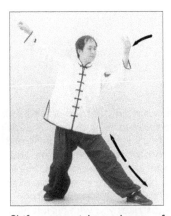 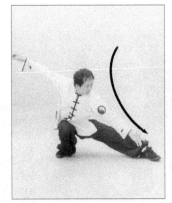

Shift your weight to the rear foot while moving your left arm back, and then lower your body as you circle your left hand down and then forward along your left leg to the foot.

Analysis:

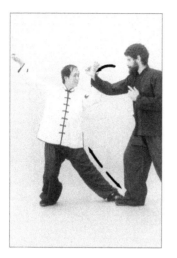 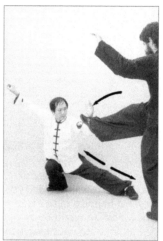

This is a defensive form that also sets the opponent up for your counterattack, for example, rooster stands on one leg (see form 31) or step forward to seven stars (see form 35). Your left hand must stick and adhere, coiling like a snake around a branch, as it leads the opponent's attacking arm into a position advantageous to you. When your opponent punches with his right hand, intercept it with your left hand and lead it to your right side. When this form is used to avoid a kick, sit back and lower your body and at the same time use your left hand to lead his kick to the side.

Cavity Strike or Striking the Vital Points

Application 1

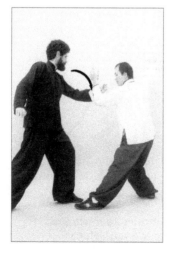

This form is mainly used to defend yourself and as a setup for your attack. The main applications will be discussed in form 31, golden rooster stands on one leg, and form 35, step forward to seven stars. Here we will limit ourselves to an example of an attack shown in the form itself. Your opponent strikes you with his left hand. Use your left hand to intercept it and guide it to the side.

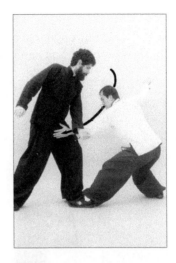

Immediately wrap your hand around his arm and move forward to attack his groin.

30. Golden Rooster Stands on One Leg (Jin Ji Du Li, 金雞獨立)

The Chinese name of this form is jin ji du li. The usual translation is correct. When a rooster stands on one leg, it is very stable and balanced. When you apply this form, you too must be balanced and stable. When you are in this stance, you can kick very easily with the lifted leg.

Movements:

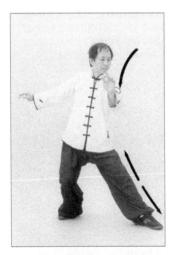

The previous form, lower the snake body, has led your opponent into a disadvantageous position.

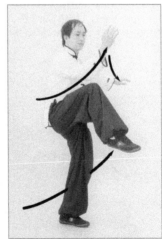

Shift your weight to your left leg and stand up, raising your right leg. When you are shifting your weight, continue to push your left hand to the side and at the same time move your right hand up to your chest.

Analysis:

Once you have sealed your opponent's attack and led his attacking hand to the side, the front of his body is exposed. You can now attack with your right hand or your right leg, or both.

Cavity Strike or Striking the Vital Points

Application 1

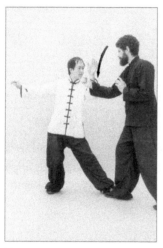
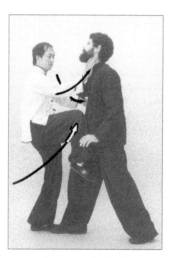

Your opponent attacks with his right hand. Use your left hand to intercept and lead it to the side.

Immediately grab his throat with your right hand and at the same time kick his dan tian with your right knee.

Application 2

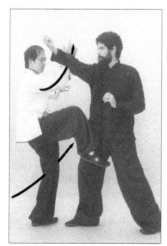

This form can also be used by itself without using the previous form, lower the snake body. Deflect your opponent's attack upward with your right arm and simultaneously kick his groin with your right leg.

31. White Snake Turns Body and Spits Poison (Bai She Tu Xin, 白蛇吐信)

The Chinese name of this form is bai she tu xin. Bai she means white snake, tu means spits, and xin means truth or a pledge—and here means poison. When a snake spits poison, it must use speed and surprise to hit its target.

Movements:

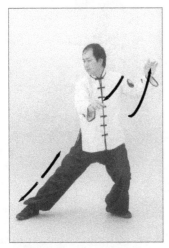
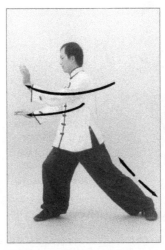

Shift about 60 percent of your weight to your left leg while twisting your body to your left and deflecting downward with your right arm.

Next turn to the right and shift your weight to the lead leg, and push your right arm to the side and your left hand forward.

Analysis:

When your opponent grabs or strikes your back, turn your body and sit back to evade the attack and expose his cavities. Shift your weight forward and attack. The strike must be fast for this form to be effective.

Cavity Strike or Striking the Vital Points

Application 1

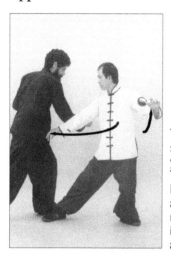

Your opponent strikes or grabs your back. Twist your body suddenly and use your right hand to intercept his arm.

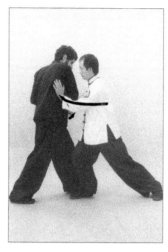

Immediately use your left hand to strike under his armpit.

32. Cross Hands (Shi Zi Shou, 十字手)

The Chinese name of this form is shi zi shou. Shi means ten, zi means word, and shou means hands. The accurate translation of this form would be "the word 'ten' hands." The Chinese character for ten is drawn with two lines intersecting to form a cross, which reflects how your hands are held in this form.

Movements:

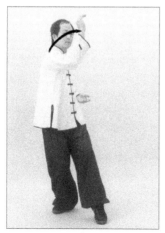

Move your right hand across your face while sitting back on your right leg, with only the toes of the left foot touching the floor.

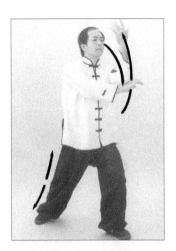

Step forward with your lead foot, continuing the motion of your right arm so that it ends horizontal in front of you, and raise your left hand vertically in front of your face.

Analysis:

You sit back to yield, and at the same time use your right hand to neutralize the opponent's attack. After neutralizing, press his arm down further to expose his face to your attack. Your left leg should be placed in an advantageous position when you step forward. While deflecting the opponent's attack, there is no weight on your left leg, and you can easily kick with it.

Downing the Enemy

Application 1

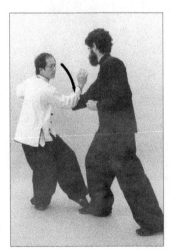

Your opponent punches with his right hand. Use your right hand to lead it to your left as you sit back.

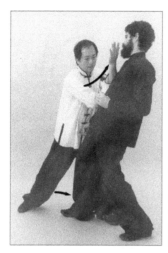

Next step your left leg behind his right leg and at the same time raise your left arm to his chest. In order to make him fall, bounce your left thigh against his leg to destroy his front root, and press his chest with your left arm and right hand.

Qin Na Control

Application 1

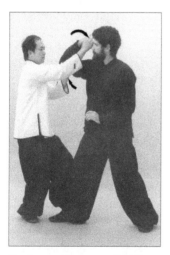

Grab your opponent's right wrist with your right hand while your left hand controls his elbow.

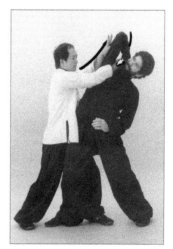

Move your right hand down and push your left hand up to control his right arm.

Cavity Strike or Striking the Vital Points

Application 1

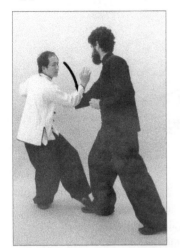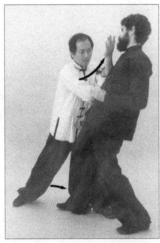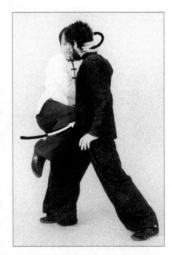

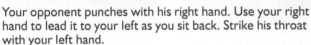

Your opponent punches with his right hand. Use your right hand to lead it to your left as you sit back. Strike his throat with your left hand.

You can also kick his groin with your right knee.

33. Brush Knee and Punch Down (Lou Xi Zhi Dang Chui, 摟膝指襠捶)

This form is called lou xi zhi dang chui in Chinese. Lou xi means to embrace the knee, zhi means finger or to aim, dang means the seat of a pair of trousers and refers to the groin area, and chui means punch. The name therefore tells you that this form is designed for brushing the opponent's kick out of the way and punching his groin. This form is very similar to form 25, step forward and strike down with the fist, the difference being that this form is for long-range fighting while the other form is for shorter-range fighting.

Movements:

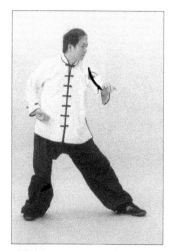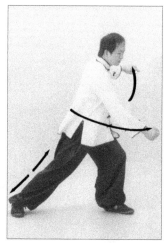

Sit back to avoid your opponent's kick, simultaneously deflecting with your left hand. Next shift your weight forward and strike down with your right hand.

Analysis:

You cannot use your hand to block a hard kick because you might break your arm. You must sit back to yield and use your hand to gently connect to his leg and lead it to the side. This exposes your opponent's groin to your punch.

Downing the Enemy

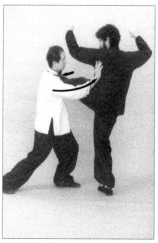

Your opponent kicks with his left leg. Sit back to yield, deflecting the kick with your left hand and extending it to your left, and then push him away with your right hand.

Cavity Strike or Striking the Vital Points

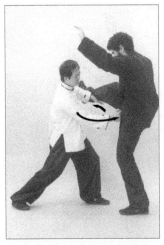 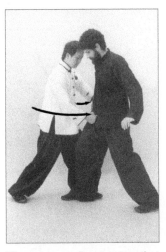

Your opponent kicks with his right leg. Sit back to yield. Use your left hand to lead his leg to your left and immediately punch his groin.

The same application can also be used when your opponent punches instead of kicks.

34. Step Forward to Seven Stars (Shang Bu Qi Xing, 上步七星)

The Chinese name of this form is shang bu qi xing. Shang bu means step forward, and qi xing means seven stars. In China, the seven stars refer to the seven stars of the Big Dipper. In this form your body resembles the constellation. Your front leg is the handle, and your body and arms the bowl. Chinese people believe that the arrangement of the seven stars hides many fighting strategies. For example, qi xing zhen (七星陣), which means seven-star tactics, refers to ways of positioning and moving troops in battle. Qi xing bu means seven-star steps (七星步) and refers to ways of stepping and moving in combat. Qi xing is also used to refer to the cavities located on the chest. In this form you step forward to form the qi xing form and strike your opponent's solar plexus area.

Movements:

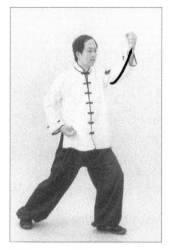 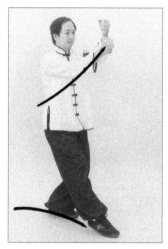

Shift your weight to your front foot and raise your left hand.

Next step your right leg forward, touching the floor with only your toes, and punch forward with your right hand.

Analysis:

Your left hand leads the opponent's arm upward to expose his chest to your right punch and his groin to a kick from your right leg.

Cavity Strike or Striking the Vital Points

Application 1

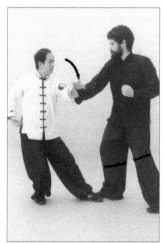

Your opponent punches with his right hand. Use your left hand to lead it down to your right.

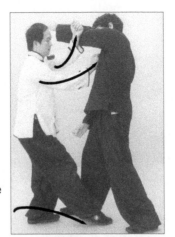

This will expose your face to his left hand. If he punches, raise your left hand to lead his attack up, and at the same time punch with your right hand to his solar plexus while stepping forward with your right leg.

Application 2

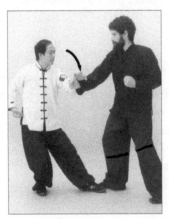
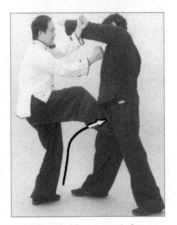

Your opponent punches with his right hand. Use your left hand to lead it down to your right. Your right foot is not weighted, so it can be used to kick the opponent's groin.

35. Step Back to Ride the Tiger (Tui Bu Kua Hu, 退步跨虎)

The Chinese name of this form is tui bu kua hu. Tui bu means step back; kua means to straddle, to encroach upon, or to pass over; and hu is tiger. This form can be translated as either "step back to ride the tiger" or "step back to pass over the tiger." The tiger is a very powerful and violent animal. If you desire to ride one, you had better hold on tightly to the hair on his back; otherwise, you will fall and become his victim. If you want to pass over a sleeping tiger, you must also be careful not to touch the tiger and wake him. Generally speaking, this form implies that your hands hold on to the opponent, and your steps should be careful to set up the most advantageous position for yourself.

Movements:

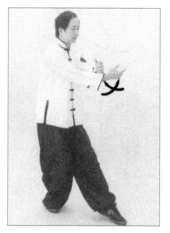 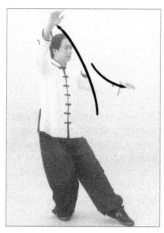

Cross both hands in front of your body while sitting back on your right leg.

Next open both hands—one up and one down.

Analysis:

This form is commonly used when your opponent grabs your lapels with the intention of pulling you down or lifting you up. You must first increase your stability by sitting back as if you are riding a tiger—firm and stable. In addition, you must grasp the opponent's arm tightly like you would hold on to the hair on the tiger's back. This will stop his attack. If, when your opponent grabs your chest, you sit back and also pull his arms toward you, you will be able to pull him off balance.

Cavity Strike or Striking the Vital Points

Application 1

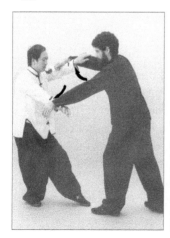

Your opponent grabs your chest or strikes you with both hands. Sit back and separate his arms with both hands.

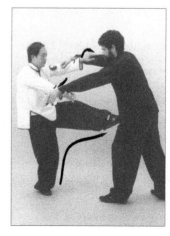

You can then kick his groin with your left leg.

36. Turn Body and Sweep Lotus (Zhuan Shen Bai Lian, 轉身擺蓮)

The Chinese name of this form is zhuan shen bai lian. Zhuan shen means to turn the body and bai lian is to sweep the lotus. There are three kicks in this form: one forward kick and two sweeping kicks. The lotus is very common in China, and children will often play at sweeping the lotus flower, which can grow fairly tall. The stem is flexible, so in order to break the stem with a sweep kick, the kick must be high, fast, and powerful.

Movements:

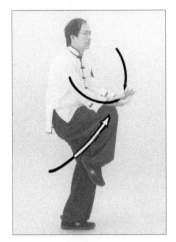

Scoop your hands down and at the same time raise your right knee.

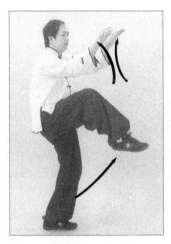

Next spread open both hands and kick forward with your right foot.

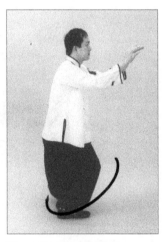

Next place your right leg behind your left leg.

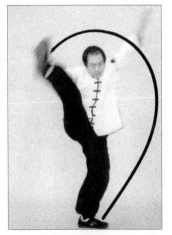

Turn and kick with your right leg in a clockwise sweep.

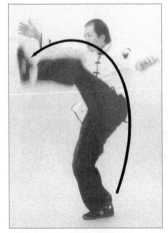

Right after the right foot touches the floor, sweep with your left leg, also in a clockwise direction.

Analysis:

There are three kicks involved in this form: a heel or toe kick, and two high sweep kicks. When kicking high, it is very important to have a firm root, for without stability, you are lost. When kicking high, you must kick very fast, because when you raise your leg, your lower body is exposed to attack, especially to sweeps and groin attacks.

Cavity Strike or Striking the Vital Points

Application 1

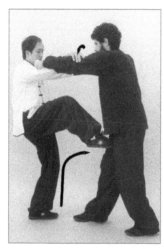

Your opponent grabs your chest. Spread your hands and grasp his arms, and at the same time kick his groin with your right leg.

Application 2

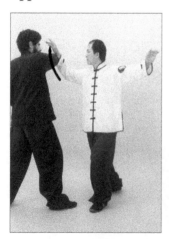

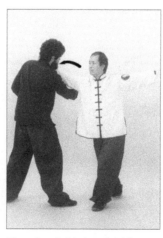

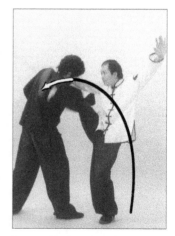

Your opponent grabs or punches you from the rear. Turn and use your right hand to deflect the attack.

Next hook his head with your right hand.

Sweep his head with your right leg.

Application 3

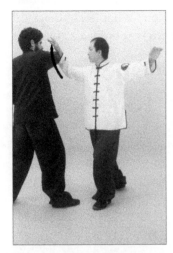

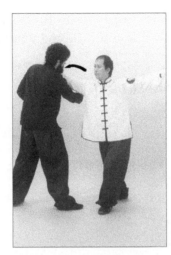

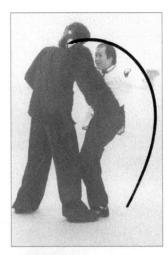

Your opponent grabs or punches you from the rear. Turn and use your right hand to deflect the attack.

Next hook his head with your right hand.

Use your left leg to sweep-kick his head.

37. Draw the Bow and Shoot the Tiger (Wan Gong She Hu, 彎弓射虎)

The Chinese name of this form is wan gong she hu. Wan gong means to bend a bow, and she hu means to shoot a tiger. When a bow is bent, it stores energy. When the arrow is shot, it is fast and powerful. This tells you that you must first store jing in your posture, and when you strike, the strike must be fast. In this form, your right hand is shaped like a bow and your left arm is like an arrow.

Movements:

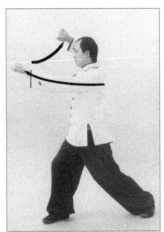

Step backward with your left leg while deflecting upward with your right hand and punching forward with your left fist.

Analysis:

Your right hand is used for deflecting and the left one for punching. Step backward as your arms move. This not only helps you yield and adjust distance, but it also balances your speed and jing.

Cavity Strike or Striking the Vital Points

Application 1

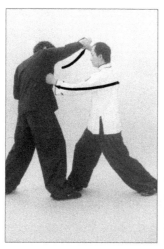

Your opponent punches you with his right hand. Deflect the attack upward with your right hand and punch under his armpit with your left hand.

The reader should understand that the applications and techniques discussed above just touch on the possibilities available in the taijiquan sequence. Once you understand all these applications, you should continue your research, pondering, and studying, and humbly ask other people for their ideas. That is the path to excellence.

Chapter 3: Taiji Pushing Hands

3-1. Introduction

Almost every Chinese martial style, both external and internal, has its own hand-matching training similar to taijiquan's pushing hands. In southern external styles, it is commonly called bridge hands (qiao shou, 橋手) or coiling hands (pan shou, 盤手). In northern external styles it is called folding hands (da shou, 搭手) or opposing hands (dui shou, 對手). Although the names are different, the purposes are the same. The techniques trained and emphasized by each style reflect the essence of that style and are usually kept secret to prevent other styles from copying them or learning how to counter them. Once a student is accepted as a legitimate student and is taught these exercises, he has begun the serious study of his style.

In taijiquan, there are also many styles of pushing hands (tui shou, 推手), because almost every different taijiquan style has its own emphasis. Some styles are extremely soft and, therefore, emphasize only the soft jing (ruanjing, 軟勁). Other styles emphasize harder jing (yingjing, 硬勁) training, which tends to be more easily accepted by beginners. Some styles stress high postures and a small defensive circle while others emphasize low postures and a large circle. Even within the same taijiquan style, there are often differences from master to master, according to their emphasis and understanding.

You may start pushing hands any time after you finish learning the solo sequence, and it should be part of your training for as long as you practice taijiquan. You learn to sense and follow your partner without resisting, so that you ultimately understand his strength and use it against him. Pushing hands also gives you a chance to practice the applications of the techniques, which increases your understanding of the sequence. Without such understanding, the sequence remains dead.

Doing taijiquan without pushing hands is like buying a car and not learning how to drive. Pushing hands teaches you how to drive in a parking lot. However, even if you can drive skillfully in this lot, it does not mean you are capable of driving on the freeway or in the city. In order to be able to "drive in real traffic," you must also learn the two-person fighting set and free fighting. The fighting set was designed to give fighting experience that resembles real fighting. This is like driving your car with an instructor's supervision. The last stage, free fighting, is your solo driving in traffic.

In pushing hands, the first step is to build up your sensitivity in the sensing jing—listening jing (tingjing, 聽勁) and understanding jing (dongjing, 懂勁). These two jing are the foundation of all taijiquan martial techniques and are developed through the practice of adhere-stick jing (zhannianjing, 粘黏勁). Until you can "hear" and understand the opponent's jing, you will not be able to understand his intention and power, and will not be able to fight effectively.

After you have grasped the tricks of listening and understanding jing, the next step is to learn how to neutralize, lead, and control the opponent's jing. Once this is learned, you will be able to react with the various offensive jing as appropriate to the situation. Naturally, during all your practice, you should not forget the fundamentals, such as keeping your body centered, comfortable, and steady, otherwise you will lose your balance. You must also remember to coordinate your qi with your jing.

In section 3 we will discuss the sounds heng (哼) and ha (哈). These are very important in taijiquan martial applications, and play a major role in raising the spirit of vitality (jing shen, 精神) and stimulating the qi to reach further and increase in strength.

Section 4 will discuss taiji ball training, which is often used in the internal styles to train listening and understanding jing. It is also used to train adhering and sticking while doing the circular advancing and retreating motions that are required in the internal martial arts.

Section 5 will discuss pushing hands. In this section the author will first introduce several basic exercises that are the key to the door of the secret of pushing hands. They will help you to understand and develop your skill at listening, understanding, and especially neutralizing (huajing, 化勁) and leading jing (yinjing, 引勁). Once you have mastered all of these basic exercises, you should practice the techniques corresponding to the eight directions, and learn how to coordinate them with your footwork according to the principles of the five elements and the eight trigrams. With this training you will be able to understand the principles and general rules of pushing hands and lay a foundation that will enable you to research and study further.

Finally, numerous examples of the martial applications of pushing-hands techniques will be discussed in section 6. These will build a foundation that will allow you to profit from the fighting set that will be discussed in the next chapter.

3-2. Key Points in Pushing-Hands Training

There are a number of important principles you should always remember and follow when practicing pushing hands. We will review these important keys in this section. If you are interested in studying in more detail some ancient documents pertaining to taijiquan, you may refer to appendix A of the book *Tai Chi Chuan Martial Power: Advanced Yang Style*, 3rd edition, by YMAA Publication Center (www.ymaa.com).

Key Points of Pushing Hands

1. The xin (heart, mind) is quiet (calm).

   Use the xin [heart, mind] to transport the qi, [the mind] must be sunk [steady] and calm, then [the qi] can condense [deep] into the bones.

   以心行氣，務令沈著，乃能收斂入骨。

2. The body is agile.

   Once in motion, every part of the body is light and agile and must be threaded together.

   一舉動，週身俱要輕靈，尤須貫穿。

3. Qi condenses.

   [The mind] leads the qi flowing back and forth, adhering to the back, then condensing into the spine; strengthen the Spirit of Vitality [Jing Shen] internally, and express externally peacefully and easily.

   牽動往來氣貼背，而練入脊骨，內固精神，外示安逸。

4. Jing is integrated and balanced.

   The root is at the feet, [jing is] generated from the legs, controlled by the waist and expressed by the fingers. From the feet to the legs to the waist must be integrated, and one unified qi. When moving forward or backward, you can then catch the opportunity and gain the superior position.

   其根在腳，發於腿，主宰於腰，形於手指。由腳而腿而腰，總須完整一氣。向前退後，乃能得機得勢。

5. Spirit is retained.

   Shen [spirit] should be retained internally.

   神宜內斂。

6. Qi must be full, stimulated, and sunken to the dan tian.

   Qi should be full and stimulated.

   氣宜鼓盪。

An insubstantial energy leads the head upward. The qi is sunk to the dan tian.

虛領頂勁， 氣沈丹田。

7. Qi must circulate freely and reach every place in the body.

Circulate the qi throughout the body, it [qi] must be smooth and fluid, then it can easily follow the mind.

以氣運身， 務令順遂， 乃能便利從心。

Transport qi as though through a pearl with a "nine-curved hole," not even the tiniest place won't be reached.

行氣如九曲珠, 無微不到。

8. Movements are continuous and not broken.

No part should be defective, no part should be deficient or excessive, no part should be disconnected.

無使有缺陷處， 無使有凸凹處， 無使有續斷處。

Step like a cat walks; applying jing is like drawing silk from a cocoon.

邁步如貓行， 運勁如抽絲。

9. The root is firm.

[If] the bubbling well [yongquan cavity] has no root, the waist has no master, [then] you can try hard to learn until you almost die, you will still not succeed.

湧泉無根， 腰無主， 力學垂死終無補。

10. The waist is loose and leads the hands.

The qi is like a cartwheel, the waist is like an axle.

氣如車輪， 腰似車軸。

In every movement the heart [mind] remains on the waist, the abdomen is relaxed and clear, and qi rises up.

刻刻留心在腰間， 腹內鬆淨氣騰然。

11. Breathing and the heng-ha sounds coordinate with the movements.

Grasp and hold the dan tian to train internal gongfu. Heng, ha, two qis are marvelous and infinite.

拿住丹田練內功， 哼哈二氣妙無窮。

12. Develop a sense of enemy.

Touch [find] the movement in the stillness, [although there is] stillness even in movement. Vary [your] response to the enemy and show the marvelous technique.

靜中觸動動猶靜， 應敵變化示神奇。

13. Do not resist. Adhere-connect, stick-follow.

When the opponent is hard, I am soft; this is called yielding. When I follow the opponent, this is called sticking.

人剛我柔謂之走， 我順人背謂之黏。

When the opponent moves fast, I move fast; when the opponent moves slowly, then I follow slowly. Although the variations are infinite, the principle remains the same.

動急則急應， 動緩則緩隨， 雖變化萬端， 而理為一貫。

When there is pressure on the left, the left becomes insubstantial; when there is pressure on the right, the right becomes insubstantial. Looking upward it seems to get higher and higher; looking downward it seems to get deeper and deeper. When [the opponent] advances, it seems longer and longer; when [the opponent] retreats, it becomes more and more urgent. A feather cannot be added and a fly cannot land. The opponent does not know me, but I know the opponent. A hero has no equal because of all of this.

左重則左虛， 右重則右杳。仰之則彌高， 俯之則彌深， 進之則愈長， 退之則愈促， 一羽不能加， 蠅蟲不能落， 人不知我， 我獨知人， 英雄所向無敵， 蓋由此而及也。

14. Footwork coordinates with the fighting strategy.

Steps change following the body.

步隨身換。

15. Distinguish substantial and insubstantial.

If there is a top, there is a bottom; if there is a front, there is a back; if there is a left, there is a right.

有上即有下，有前即有後，有左即有右。

Substantial and insubstantial must be clearly distinguished. Every part [of the body] has a substantial and an insubstantial aspect. The entire body and all the joints should be threaded together without the slightest break.

虛實宜分清楚，一處有一處虛實，處處總此皆如是。周身節節貫串，無令絲毫間斷耳。

16. The body is upright and centered.

No tilting, no leaning.

不偏不倚。

Stand like a balanced scale, [move] lively like a cartwheel.

立如平準，活似車輪。

When standing, the body must be centered, calm and comfortable, so you can handle the eight directions.

立身須中正安舒支撐八面。

There are three selections from the *Taijiquan Classics* that are concerned specifically with pushing hands. They have been included along with commentary in appendix A of the book *Tai Chi Chuan Martial Power: Advanced Yang Style*, from YMAA Publication Center.

Song of Eight Words

Wardoff [peng], rollback [lu], press [ji], and push [an] are rare in this world. Ten martial artists, ten don't know. If [you are] able to be light and agile, also strong and hard, [then you gain] adhere-connect, stick-follow with no doubt. Pluck [cai], split [lie], elbow stroke [zhou], and shoulder stroke [kao] are even more remarkable. When used, no need to bother your mind. If you gain the secret of the words adhere-connect, stick-follow, then you will be in the ring and not scattered.

掤、搌、擠、按世界稀， 十個藝人十不知。若能輕靈並堅硬， 沾、連、黏、隨俱無疑。
採、挒\肘、靠更出奇， 行之不用費心思。果得沾、連、黏、隨字， 得其環中不支離。

Song of Pushing Hands

Be conscientious about wardoff [peng], rollback [lu], press [ji], and push [an]. Up and down follow each other, [then] the opponent [will find it] difficult to enter.

掤、搌、擠、按須認真， 上下相隨人難進。

No matter [if] he uses enormous power to attack me, [I] use four ounces to lead [him aside], deflecting [his] one thousand pounds.

任他巨力來打我， 牽動四兩撥千斤。

Guide [his power] to enter into emptiness, then immediately attack; adhere-connect, stick-follow, do not lose him.

引進落空合即出， 沾、連、黏、隨不丟頂。

The Secret of Withdraw and Release

First Saying: Deflect

Deflect and open opponent's body and borrow opponent's li [strength].

一曰擎， 擎開彼身借彼力。

Second Saying: Lead

Lead [opponent's power] near [my] body, jing thereby stored.

二曰引， 引到身前勁始蓄。

Third Saying: Relax

Relax and expand my jing, without bends.

三曰鬆， 鬆開我勁勿使屈。

Fourth Saying: Release

When [I] release, the waist and the feet must be timed carefully and accurately.

四曰放， 放時腰腳認端的。

3-3. Heng and Ha Sounds

In this section, we will discuss the methods of heng (哼) and ha (哈) sounds training. But first, let us review their yin-yang relationship.

The Heng Sound. There are two ways to make the heng sound. The first is when you are exhaling while making the sound; the sound is classified as positive (yang) but with some yin. It is used when you are making an attack and you do not want the jing completely out. This is commonly used with yang jing that have some yin. The second heng sound is made when you are inhaling. In this case, it is purely yin and is used when you are neutralizing, yielding, or retreating. When this sound is made, your spirit is focused and your qi is condensed deep into the bones to store energy.

The Ha Sound. The ha sound is pure yang and thus positive. This sound is commonly used when you are using pure yang jing to attack the opponent. This sound will raise your spirit of vitality (jing shen, 精神) to its maximum and enable your qi to support the jing most effectively while attacking.

To practice the heng-ha sounds, stand with the feet a comfortable distance apart. Even though the sounds can be made silently, it is best to start doing the ha sound as a loud yell and the heng sound as a quieter exhalation or inhalation with some sound coming from the larynx. When practicing, remember the following important points:

1. Yi Is Extended and Concentrated

When these sounds are made, your yi (mind) must be farther than the target in order to lead the qi to flow without any stagnation or hesitation. For example, when you make the ha sound in attacking the opponent, your yi must be inside your opponent's body, and then you will be able to lead your qi to the palm to support your attacking jing. Similarly, when you make an inhaling heng sound, your yi must be deep in your marrow in order to lead the qi to condense there. Not only should your yi be extended, but it must also be focused and concentrated, otherwise your qi, and therefore your jing, will be scattered and weak. In training the heng and ha sounds, your yi should be focused as far away and deeply as possible. Then, when you need to use your qi, it will be strong, and you will be able to extend it into your arms or weapon to support your jing. For example, when you use a weapon such as a sword or a spear for attacking, your yi and qi must reach to the end of the weapon. Without extension and focus training, your weapon techniques will not be effective or powerful.

2. Qi Is Balanced, Full, and Extended

When you utter the heng or ha sounds, you should always seek to extend and balance your qi, and to have it completely fill your body. When you make the ha sound, you should direct a flow of qi in the direction the sound is moving, and a second flow of qi to the dan tian and down to the feet. The qi stored in the dan tian must be full and stimulated. In order to do this, the yi must be condensed, and the breathing must be deep. This will also enable the qi that flows upward to extend farther. When inhaling with the heng sound, condense your spirit and your yi and lead your qi to the spine and marrow. At the same time, lead the qi from the bottom of your feet up to the dan tian. When the exhaling heng sound is made, the qi balance is the same as with the ha sound but with one difference: the exhaling heng sound holds part of the qi at the dan tian.

3. The Sound Is Focused and Condensed

The sounds should be focused and condensed, but this will only happen if your yi and qi are focused and condensed. The sounds come from the dan tian and not from the throat, and they are strong, solid, and extended.

4. Hand Forms

The hands are where you sense and attack the opponent. Therefore, the final goal of sound training is to enable you to lead qi to your palms and even farther to your weapons. When you exhale, especially with the ha sound, you should feel a strong flow of qi to your palms, which you may perceive as warmth and tingling. When inhaling with the heng sound, you should sense your qi flowing back to your body, to the spine and dan tian. There are a few hand forms that are useful in training the heng-ha sounds. The beginner should hold his hands lightly over his dan tian when practicing so that he can more easily sense and control the in-and-out motion of the dan tian. The abdomen around the dan tian should expand when you exhale and withdraw when you inhale. Once you can coordinate this naturally, you can use the different hand forms to lead the qi to your palms or withdraw it from them.

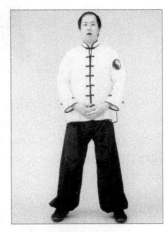

Beginner hand form.

The ha sound is yang and purely positive, and you should use an open hand form. The open hand form is yang and positive, and all the qi extends outward through the palms and fingers. When you practice, hold your palms face down in front of your waist. Alternatively, you may extend your hands in front of your chest with your palms facing forward.

The exhaled heng sound is yang with some yin, so you should use different hand forms. Touch your thumb with either your index finger or middle finger so that part of the qi flows out and part of it recirculates back through the touch-

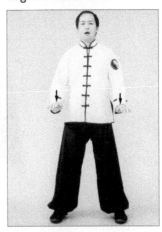

Open hand form for ha sound.

ing fingers. As when practicing the ha sounds, you may place your hands in front of either your waist or your chest.

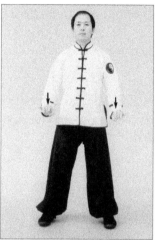

Hand form for exhaled heng sound.

The inhaled heng sound is pure yin and negative, and helps the qi flow back to the body and condense into the bones. As you practice this sound, the extended fingers should gently curve in, and at the same time you should raise them somewhat if you are holding them in front of your waist or draw your hands back toward your shoulders if they are extended out.

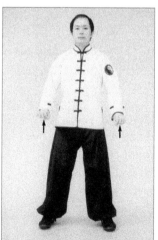

Hand form for inhaled heng sound.

The inhaled heng sound is usually practiced together with the exhaled ha. There are several ways your hands can help your visualization.

Method 1: Start with the hands in front of your waist. Slightly raise both hands palm up for the inhalation, then turn your palms down and press downward for the exhaled ha sound. You should have a feeling of raising your spirit of vitality and condensing your qi into your spine when you inhale with the heng sound. When you make the ha sound, the qi sinks, your root is strengthened, and at the same time your qi is transported through your extremities and to your skin.

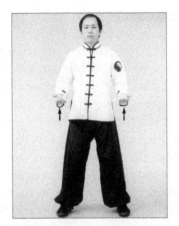 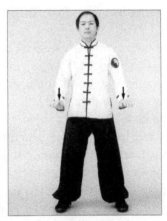

Inhaled heng sound and exhaled ha sound, method 1.

Method 2: Hold your hands in front of your chest. As you inhale with the heng sound, draw your hands in toward your chest as your fingers come together. As you exhale with the ha sound, push your open palms forward. While making the heng sound, condense your qi into your spine, and while making the ha sound, lead the qi to your palms.

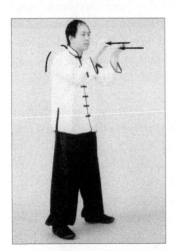 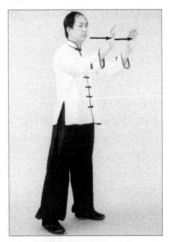

Inhaled heng sound and exhaled ha sound, method 2.

When you have practiced these sounds a bit, it doesn't mean that you can use them effectively in a fight. In a fight, your yi of sound and yi of qi must be one unit. This means that there should be only one yi that should raise your spirit of vitality and lead your qi to the desired place at the same time. In order to do this, you must practice them in pushing hands and the two-person fighting set so that you naturally use them correctly without thinking.

3-4. Taiji Ball Training

Taiji ball has been commonly used for training in the internal martial styles developed in the Wudang (武當) and Emei (峨嵋) mountains. It is an effective tool for leading the taijiquan beginner into the world of pushing hands. The ball can be used by beginners to learn several important fundamental jing and by the advanced student to train special jing. This training can be solo or with a partner. It is also commonly used to exercise the hands and arms to generate local qi, which benefits the health. In the last fifty years, the taiji ball has been neglected, and many training methods have been forgotten. The author hopes this section will encourage the reader to practice and research this almost-lost art. Taiji ball training is good for the health as well as the martial arts. If you are interested in knowing more about taiji ball qigong, please refer to the book *Tai Chi Ball Qigong: For Health and Martial Arts* and the DVDs *Tai Chi Ball Qigong: Courses 1 and 2*, by YMAA Publication Center (www.ymaa.com).

In taijiquan, several jing form the foundation of the art. These are listening jing (tingjing, 聽勁), understanding jing (dongjing, 懂勁), and adhere-stick jing (zhannianjing, 粘黏勁). Without the first two jing, an internal-style fighter would be like a blind person walking a rocky, uneven road. With no adhere-stick capability, he would be like a sword fighter without a sword. Taiji ball has also been used by advanced practitioners to develop a higher level of adhere-stick jing called pan-xi jing (coil-suction jing, 盤吸勁). When someone skilled in this jing touches you, you feel like he is glued to you and you cannot pull away. It is an aggressive and active aspect of adhere-stick jing.

The Ball

The ball can be as small as a ping-pong ball to train the fingers in listening and understanding jing, or it can be as big as two feet in diameter for the advanced practitioner to train coil-suction jing. The most common and useful size for a beginner is about a foot in diameter—about the size of a basketball. The surface should be as smooth as possible, and the material should not be plastic. Wood is the best material, and the ideal weight is three to five pounds. To prevent cracking due to changes in the weather, the surface should be coated with varnish, or the ball should be soaked in vegetable oil. A solid or hollow metal ball is not good for practice, not only because of the heavy weight, but mainly because the metal ball will absorb the qi from your skin, which will significantly reduce your qi control and sensitivity.

Where to Practice

The most comfortable way to practice is on a table or other flat surface about the height of your waist.

Areas of the Body to Train

The main areas of your body that you use in training with the taiji ball are the places that most commonly touch the opponent in a fight: the fingers, palms, back of the hands, wrists, forearms, and elbows.

General Principles of Training

1. Movement from the Body

It is a basic principle of taijiquan that the hands do not move by themselves; rather, the motion comes from the body. Use your waist to lead your arms to move the ball.

2. Relaxed and Light Contact

To increase the sensitivity of your listening, your muscles must be relaxed to allow the qi to circulate. Contact must be light and easy. If your contact is heavy, your muscles will interfere with the qi circulation, and your sensitivity will be limited. If you cannot listen well, your understanding will be limited, and you will not be able to adhere and stick effectively.

3. Yi Is Concentrated

When you practice taiji ball, your yi must be calm and concentrated on your sense of touch. Your yi leads your qi; if your yi is scattered, your qi will not flow smoothly. Yi also plays a main role in understanding, because if you listen without really concentrating your mind, you will not understand what you hear.

4. Breathing Coordinates with Your Movements

Just as in other aspects of taijiquan training, breathing plays an important role in leading qi to the area desired. Therefore, when you practice taiji ball, inhale to take in qi from the ball, and exhale to push your qi into the ball.

5. From Slow to Fast

As with the solo sequence, practice slowly at first. As your skill increases, gradually increase your speed to shorten the time you have for listening, understanding, adhering, and sticking. This will keep the training alive and active, and help you develop agility in pushing hands and free fighting.

Taiji Ball Training

1. Circling and Squaring

Circling is the foundation and basic principle of taijiquan. Therefore, first build up your sensitivity and the spiritual correspondence between you and the ball by moving the ball in circles with your palm.

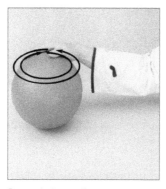 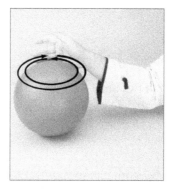

Start with small circles, using the center or the edge of your palm, then gradually start using the back of your hand, wrist, forearm, and elbow. When you can circle smoothly without losing touch with the ball, increase the size of your circles.

You will notice that the larger circles are harder to do. They require fairly good listening, understanding, and adhere-stick jing to keep circling smoothly and to maintain contact with the ball. When the diameter of the circle increases to about the diameter of the ball itself, you must have coil-suction jing to keep control of the ball. This is a very high level of taiji ball training.

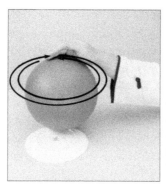

The next stage of practice is to place a plate upside down on the table and repeat the above training with the ball on the plate. This is much harder.

When you practice directly on the table, it is easy to find the centerline that allows you to sense the root of the ball. However, when you practice on a plate, the plate can move, and it is easy to lose control of the ball. You must really develop your understanding jing to be able to sense the root of the plate through the root of the ball, and to circle the ball without moving the plate. The highest level of this practice is to circle your taiji ball on top of other balls of various sizes.

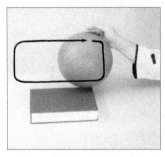

You can also do these exercises on a square or rectangular object, such as a book, by moving your ball around the outside edge of the object.

The lighter the object, the harder it will be. The final goal of this practicing is to develop the capacity to trace any object without moving it. Closing your eyes as you practice helps you develop your sensitivity more quickly.

2. Forward, Backward, and Sideways

In addition to circling, you should also practice moving the ball forward and backward as well as sideways. The training principle is the same, but this time, you move the ball in a straight line or perhaps a curved line.

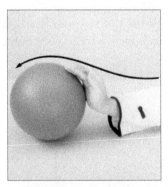 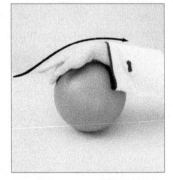

An example of this practice is pushing forward with the edge of your palm and guiding the ball backward with your fingers.

3. Coil-Suction Jing (盤吸勁)

As mentioned, coil-suction jing is the hardest and highest level of adhere-stick jing. In addition to the abovementioned training methods, coil-suction jing can also be trained in the following way.

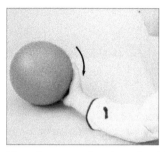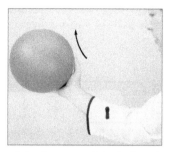

First place your hand on the side of the bottom of the ball and try to pick it up by changing the angle.

If you can pick the ball up easily, then try gradually to pick it up more and more from the side of the ball, and finally from the top of the ball. The principle of this is to place your hand flat on the ball, and then arc the center of your palm back to create a vacuum. This is the most difficult jing; even in ancient times, only a few martial artists achieved it. The best ones needed only to touch your skin to generate a vacuum. Nowadays, you can occasionally see coil-suction jing performed by Chinese acrobats or gongfu demonstrators. However, if you watch carefully, you will find that they usually need to use the other hand to hold the object firmly in the first hand before they can create a vacuum.

4. Two-Handed Practice

In pushing hands or in a real fight, you must use both of your hands effectively. Two-handed taiji ball develops skill in this mutual circling and trains your hands to coordinate with and assist each other.

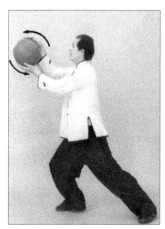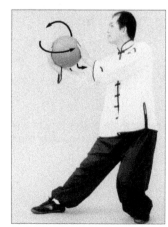

Circling forward.

Circling backward.

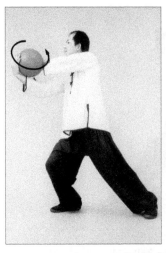

Sideward circling forward.

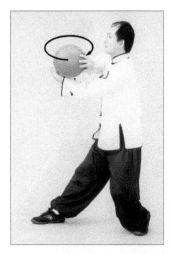

Sideward circling backward.

In all of these exercises, the legs should move in coordination with the circling and advancing and retreating strategies. Without this coordination, the techniques will be sluggish and clumsy. In this training, you should also imagine that you are pushing hands with a partner so that you can practice setting up your strategies. Without this kind of imagining, you will not be able to build up a sense of enemy, and your practice will not help you in a real fight.

A common way to practice taiji ball with two hands is to practice wardoff, rollback, press, and push.

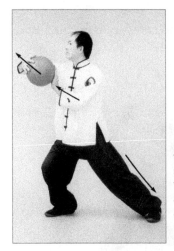

Execute wardoff slightly upward with your right arm. The left arm provides a countering support.

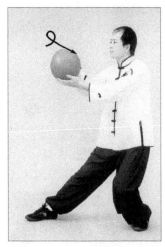

Rotate the ball and change your posture into rollback.

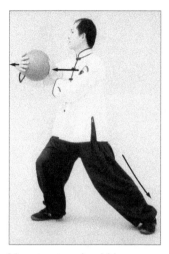 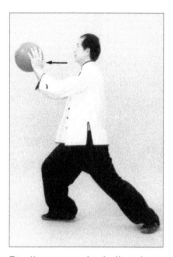

Your motion should be circular, and you should have a feeling of leading. Continue the motion and practice press. This form looks like wardoff, but there are two differences. First, the direction of press is forward instead of slightly upward. Second, the wrist is used to strike, firmly supported by your left hand.

Finally, rotate the ball and withdraw to the front of your chest, and then push forward. Practice these four basic forms repeatedly until you can do them smoothly and comfortably.

5. Two-Person Practice

Once you have mastered solo practice, you should go on to two-person practice. Both partners hold the ball with both hands.

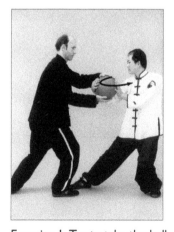 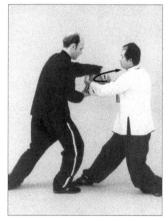

Exercise 1: Try to take the ball away from each other.

You need to have the right strategy, know the right direction, and understand your partner's jing and yi. Do not hold the ball too tightly or too loosely; imagine you are holding an egg, and you will understand. Be careful to avoid struggling with each other. Turn your body and reposition your hands so that you can slip the ball away from your partner or keep him from slipping it away from you.

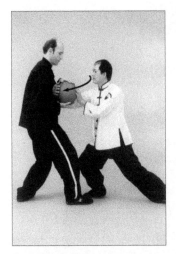 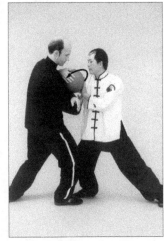 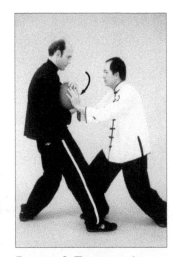

Exercise 2: Try to touch your partner's body with the back of your hand.

Exercise 3: Try to touch your partner with the ball.

Naturally, your partner will do the same to you and also try to avoid your attempts. You must be skilled in listening, understanding, and adhere-stick jing, and you must also know neutralization jing so that you can lead your partner's attacking jing into emptiness. Skill in this exercise will lay a good foundation for pushing hands.

The exercises discussed above are only some examples of taiji ball training. There are many other training methods available, and you can even create your own methods as long as they help you to train listening, understanding, and adhering-sticking.

3-5. Pushing-Hands Training

Open Doors and Windows

Before starting pushing hands, you should first understand two strategic concepts that are commonly used in Chinese martial society. The first term is called open door (kong men, 空門). An open door is a space through which you can most easily approach and attack your opponent. The principle is pretty simple: when you stand your legs give you stability and strength, but they also determine the directions in which you are weakest. While your stability is greatest along the line between your two legs, you are weakest at right angles to this line. If you are pushed or pulled in the directions in which you are weak, you will easily lose your balance and fall. The figure below shows the directions of the open doors.

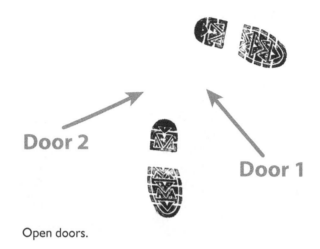

Open doors.

When your opponent is standing with his right leg forward, he has two open doors. Door 1 is called the left open door (zuo kong men, 左空門) and is the easiest one to enter or attack from. Door 2 is called the right open door (you kong men, 右空門) and is usually harder to use.

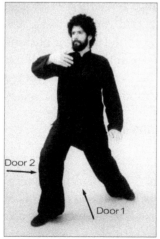

Opponent is standing with his right leg forward. Door 1 is called the left open door. Door 2 is called the right open door.

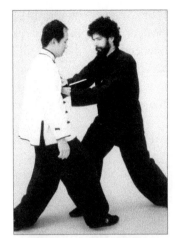 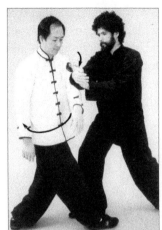

Your opponent presses your chest. You can neutralize the press to your right.

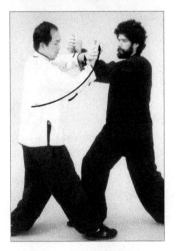 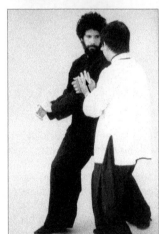

Next circle his hand to the left, step to readjust your position, and attack him from his left open door.

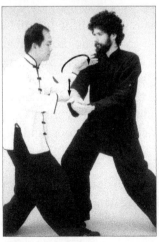 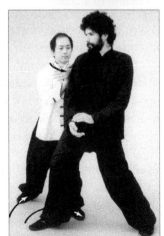

Alternatively, you can neutralize his press to your right, step to readjust your position, and press his back from his right open door. The same principle applies when your opponent is standing with the other leg forward.

The second concept is called the window (chuang, 窗). Windows are also areas through which you can attack your opponent and apply your techniques on his body. Usually, when you fight against an experienced martial artist, all his windows are closed. Therefore, you will not be able to attack through a window without exerting some effort. In order to attack through a window, you must open it and then attack immediately. Usually, you can open the opponent's window easily, but he can close it just as easily.

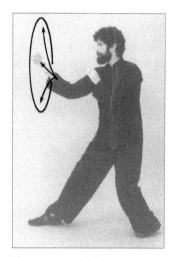

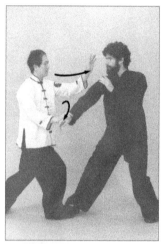

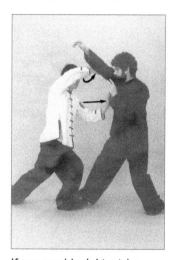

Your opponent is standing with his right leg forward and his right hand in front of his chest. His right windows are considered closed because he can use his right hand to protect the right side of his body effectively and give you no chance to attack.

However, if you have the chance to grab his right wrist with your right hand and press it down, then you have opened the sky window (tian chuang, 天窗) for your attack.

If you can block his right hand upward, you can expose his waist area for your attack. You have opened his ground window (di chuang, 地窗).

As mentioned, if your enemy is very skillful, he will be able to close his windows very fast after you have opened it and give you no chance to attack.

Once you understand the concepts of open doors and windows, you will be able to understand the principles of fighting strategy. Downing the enemy techniques depend upon your effective use of your opponent's open door, and cavity strikes are ineffective unless you know how to open the opponent's windows. The pushing-hands techniques in this chapter are based on the concepts of doors and windows.

Pushing-Hands Practice Concepts

Pushing-hands training can be divided into stationary pushing hands (ding bu tui shou, 定步推手) and moving pushing hands (dong bu tui shou, 動步推手). Normally, you start with stationary pushing hands and stay with it until you have developed a degree of listening and understanding jing. You can then add footwork in coordination with your techniques and strategies. In this section we will introduce a range of pushing-hands techniques from the most fundamental to the more advanced. Once you have mastered these techniques, you should still not be satisfied, because until you can apply them naturally and skillfully, they are all dead. Even when you can apply them easily, you are still not finished. At this stage you should research different ways to train. Innovation is the way to learn; you must create, develop, and grow. However, before you do this, you should master an existing style and its techniques.

Before you start pushing-hands training, there are a few principles (in addition to those mentioned in section 2) that you should know:

1. From Stationary to Moving

In stationary pushing-hands practice, you are always rooted, and because no steps are involved, you can concentrate all your attention on coordinating your hands and body. Also, because you cannot evade your opponent's attack by stepping, you are forced to learn how to neutralize. Only after you have mastered stationary practice should you go on to moving pushing hands.

2. From Slow to Fast

In the beginning you must practice slowly and only increase your speed when you have developed understanding and sticking and adhering jing. Starting fast is like trying to run before you have learned to walk. If you do this, you will probably miss one of the most important points in taiji pushing-hands training, which is the principle of sticking and following. Training from slow to fast also allows you to train your yi, qi, and jing gradually along with your techniques. Without yi, qi, and jing, your pushing hands will be useless and ineffective. Last, practicing from slow to fast makes it much easier to train the coordination of your breathing with the techniques.

3. From Low to High

When you first start pushing hands, your root is poor. The best way to develop your root is to practice with a low stance. In time, the muscles in your legs will be loose enough to allow the qi to flow smoothly to the bottom of your feet. Only when your yi and qi can reach the bubbling well points in your feet will you be able to build a firm root, and only then should you gradually make your posture higher and higher.

4. From Expanded to Compact

When you first start your pushing-hands training, your listening and understanding capability is still low. You should start with a large defensive circle that allows you more time and distance to sense the opponent's intention. Only after you have mastered the large defensive circle should you start to decrease the size of the circle. If you can follow this learning procedure, your taiji pushing hands will gradually develop from sluggish to smooth, from broken to connected, and from dead to alive.

This section will first discuss basic pushing-hands exercises and then eight-trigram and five-element training, and will conclude with silk-reeling exercises (Yang-style yin/yang symbol sticking hands, Chen-style Chan si jing, 纏絲勁) and bagua circle walking.

Fundamental Training of Pushing Hands

1. Listening, Understanding, Yielding, Neutralizing, and Leading
(聽、懂、讓、化、引)

In taijiquan martial applications, listening, understanding, yielding, neutralizing, and leading are probably the most important factors that decide who wins a fight. "Listening" refers to the sensing you do with your skin—your perception of the opponent's energy or qi. "Understanding" is the intuitive understanding of the opponent's intention, sometimes at the first touch. When you understand what he is attempting, you can react appropriately.

Your listening ability depends to a great degree upon your qi circulation. The more your qi can reach to your skin, the better you can sense your opponent's jing and qi. In understanding, the more you practice, the better you will be able to understand. Therefore, your listening and understanding capability comes from your accumulated pushing-hands experience and qi training.

In taijiquan, once you have come to an understanding of the opponent's intention, you can react defensively, offensively, or both. In any case, however, you must first nullify or avoid your opponent's attack. There are many jing involved in this, the most important of which are yielding, neutralizing, and leading. Normally, you "use four ounces to neutralize the opponent's one-thousand-pound attack" (四兩破千斤) and then lead his attack to where it can do you the most good. Very often, you will yield first, then neutralize, and finally lead. These are the foundations of taijiquan's pushing-hands and fighting strategy. Without this basic foundation, taijiquan loses its original principle—that of using the soft against the hard, of defeating the strong with the weak. For these reasons, before you start actual pushing hands, you should first focus on training exercises that will develop your level of listening, understanding, yielding, neutralizing, and leading.

In your entire body, your hands and arms are the most important places for listening and understanding jing. You must build your sensitivity there first, and then you can expand this listening and understanding capability to your entire body. These two jing are usually practiced together with yielding, neutralizing, and leading jing. We will first discuss the training of listening, understanding, neutralizing, and leading jing, and then the training where yielding is used before neutralizing.

Listening, Understanding, Neutralizing, and Leading

In neutralizing jing, you "use four ounces of power to neutralize one thousand pounds." In order to do this, you must use your opponent's power against him. Timing is extremely important. It is said: "The opponent does not move, I do not move; the opponent moves slightly, I move first." This means that you must neutralize when your opponent's yi is out but just before his jing comes out. Then you can use your four ounces to neutralize his one-thousand-pound attack.

Hand and Wrist Neutralization

In pushing hands, your hands and wrists are probably the most important places for neutralizing your opponent's attack. When these two places neutralize and lead correctly, your opponent's attack will be immediately nullified. These two spots are the keys to using four ounces to neutralize one thousand pounds. They are like the ring in a bull's nose that allows you to lead it wherever you want.

Generally speaking, you can neutralize an attack in any of four directions—up, down, and to either side. The trick to neutralization is rotation. When you push a ball, it rotates and neutralizes your push to the side. You too must use rotation to neutralize an attack.

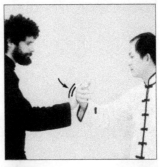

To practice with your right hand, face your partner in the mountain-climbing stance with your right foot forward. Your opponent's right hand should lightly touch your right wrist.

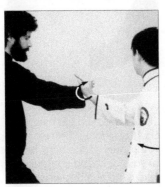

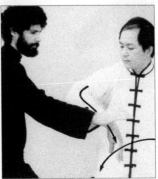

He should then press his right hand against your wrist. The direction of the press can be straight forward, slightly upward, sideward, or downward. Neutralize according to the direction he is pushing (i.e., you should generally rotate in the direction he is moving). In sideward neutralization, you rotate your wrist to the right or to the left.

Your whole body must be involved in this motion. For example, when you neutralize to the left, rotate your whole body to the left as you turn your right wrist counterclockwise. At the end of your neutralization, your right hand should be controlling his right wrist, and your forearm should be crossing his arm to control it. Remember: your waist leads the arms; it doesn't just coordinate with them.

You can also neutralize the attack upward or downward with a rotation of your wrist.

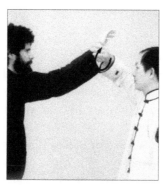

Neutralizing upward.

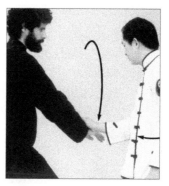

When you neutralize upward, you expose your chest. Therefore, you should also rotate your body to your right and immediately guide his wrist down and to your side.

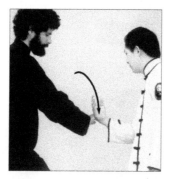

Neutralizing downward.

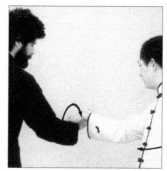

When you neutralize downward, you expose your chest to attack. Therefore, you should rotate your body to your right and immediately take control of his wrist with your hand.

Practice slowly at first, and increase the speed only after you have grasped the trick of neutralization. By this time, too, your listening and understanding capability must also be higher. At the end of your neutralization, you should be in control of your opponent's wrist. Stay attached to it, and lead it a little further in the same direction it is already moving. This will cause him to overextend and expose his vital areas to your attack. Remember: you must neutralize first, and then you can lead.

Forearm Neutralization

The same principles of rotation and leading with the waist should also be applied when using the forearm to neutralize.

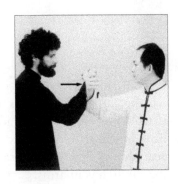

To do this exercise training your right arm, face your partner with your right foot forward in the mountain-climbing stance and your forearm lightly touching your partner's.

Either one of you uses his forearm to press the partner's forearm onto his chest. You can press straight forward, slightly upward, sideward, or downward. When you sense your opponent's attack, notice its direction, speed, and power. Once you understand the attack, you must react immediately to neutralize the pressure and lead it into emptiness. Your arm should not resist the pressure. Remain lightly touching your partner's arm, and lead all of his attacks into emptiness.

As in the previous section, your waist plays the central role when you neutralize the opponent's press to the right or left. Your waist must lead the neutralization in close coordination with the rotation of your arm.

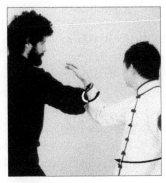

Right neutralization.

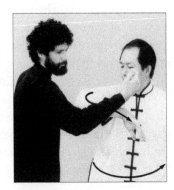

Left neutralization.

When you neutralize your opponent's press upward and downward, you should also rotate your body and also try to control his wrist immediately after the neutralization.

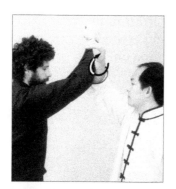 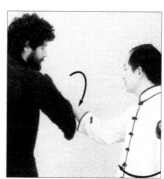

Upward neutralization.

Once you and your partner learn how to do these turning neutralizations, start an open drill where each can press the other's arm at any time. When you find that your partner's yi is scattered and his posture is advantageous to you, catch this opportunity and press him. Both of you should practice until you do not feel any resistance and all the attacks are neutralized. Then you can say that you have caught the key to listening and understanding through your arms.

As with hand and wrist neutralization training, it is best to start with slower attacks so you have time to sense them. After both of you have built up your sensitivity, increase the speed and use a stronger press jing. Train both arms, and practice with different partners so that you will get as much and as varied experience as possible. Once you have reached this level, start to practice stepping into the opponent's open door where you can most easily defeat him. This forces your opponent to adjust his position in order to neutralize your attack.

Neutralization with Yielding First

In this basic exercise, you should yield before you neutralize. The figure below shows the difference in the applications when yielding is used and when it is not. When neutralizing with the wrist or forearm, you will often find that you cannot neutralize in time and your arm is pushed against your chest. In this case you must yield first so that the attack enters into emptiness. After you have yielded to his attack, and just before his jing is completely out, neutralize his remaining jing and lead him into a disadvantageous position. Frequently, you will have to adjust your feet to make your opponent miss his target. To practice yielding before neutralizing, use the same exercises mentioned in the last section except that you now yield first until your opponent's jing is almost out, and then neutralize and lead. The simplest way to yield is to shift your weight to your rear foot as much or as little as necessary. In many cases you will have to adjust your feet by stepping either your front or your rear foot to the side or rear. Remember that you neutralize by turning your waist, not just by moving your arm.

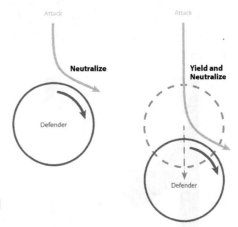

The difference in the applications when yielding is used and when it is not.

2. Controlling (Na) Training

Na (拿) is another key to winning in pushing hands. Na can put your opponent in a passive position and set him up for your attack. When na is used in qin na, it can control the opponent's joints according to the principles of dividing the muscles and misplacing the bones. When na is properly used in sticking, it can force your opponent to change his offense into defense. When sticking na is used effectively, it will make your opponent feel that you are sticking to his joints like flypaper and he cannot get rid of you. Na techniques have been regularly trained in both southern Chinese styles and some northern styles such as Tiger Claw, White Crane, and Eagle Claw.

Na in taijiquan is somewhat different from the na that is trained in external styles. Unless qin na is applied, na in taijiquan is relatively soft and relaxed compared to sticking na in external styles. In taijiquan na jing, you adhere to the opponent's joints, such as the wrist, elbow, and shoulder, in order to control his movement and immobilize any attempt to attack. The details of taijiquan na jing have been explained in the book *Tai Chi Chuan Martial Power*, 3rd edition, from YMAA Publication Center, so we will not repeat them. Here we will emphasize only the training methods and principles.

A. Wrist

When you want to control your opponent's wrist, the first consideration in almost all situations is to have your hand on top of his wrist. In this case, your opponent's arm is immobilized and loses its freedom, which gives you a chance to attack. Naturally, your opponent will attempt to free his hand and reverse the situation. Generally speaking, there are two methods of preventing this. The first way is to resist his motion for an instant when he starts to move, and the second is to use leading jing to redirect his motion either back to where it started, or else to lead it to another disadvantageous position. In either case, agilely rotate your palm, and use your four fingers to maintain your contact and control. While the thumb is sometimes used, especially when your opponent's arm is resting in the V between your thumb and forefinger, you should usually avoid using the thumb to control because it can easily get jammed and injured, and also because you will find it too easy to use force and resist.

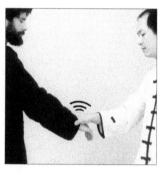

Control your opponent with your hand on top of his wrist.

There are two ways to reverse the controlling situation.

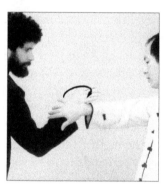 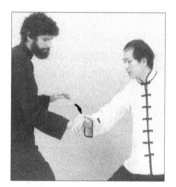

Your opponent can reverse your control from the outside of your hand.

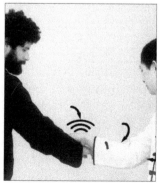

When your opponent attempts to counter from the outside of your palm, rotate your wrist so that your four fingers cover his motion.

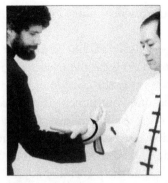 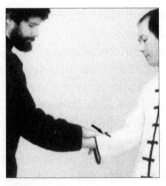

When your opponent is controlled, he can reverse your control from the inside of your hand.

If he attempts to counter from your thumb side, rotate your hand so that your four fingers can again suppress his motion and control him. If he attempts to pull his hand back from your control, follow his pull and take the opportunity to attack him.

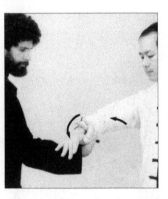

Practice with your right hand against your opponent's right wrist, your left against his left, and also your left hand against his right wrist and your right against his left. After you have mastered single-hand control training, then practice controlling both of your opponent's wrists at the same time.

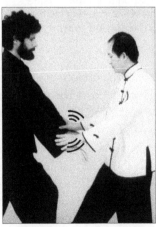

Practice controlling both of your opponent's wrists at the same time.

In this wrist-controlling training, you should also learn how to counter the opponent's na to your wrist.

Remember that in this situation, your elbow functions like your waist in that it generates the turning and coiling jing that you use to reverse the situation. In double-hand na training, the situation can be reversed from either the outside or the inside. You can prevent your opponent from doing this by rotating your hands. The figure below shows black trying to reverse the situation from the outside and white rotating his hands to the outside to stop him. Following the same principle, the next figure shows black trying from the inside and white rotating his hands inside to stop the attempt. Your opponent may also try one hand outside and one hand inside, but the principle remains the same, and you neutralize each hand individually. Remember that when you counter, your elbows are down and your body sunk. The motion is relaxed and fast, but muscle usage is cut down to its minimum.

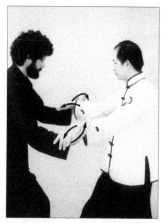

Black trying to reverse the situation from the outside, and white rotating his hands to the outside to stop him.

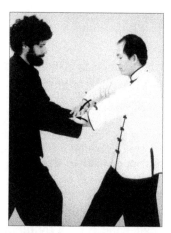

Black trying from the inside, and white rotating his hands inside to stop the attempt.

B. Elbow

When you control the opponent's wrist, he can still use his elbow to strike you. When you control his elbow, he loses the use of both his elbow and hand; however, he can still use his shoulder to strike you. Generally speaking, controlling the wrist is easier than controlling the elbow, and controlling the elbow is easier than controlling the shoulder. To control your opponent's elbow, lead or press it upward or sideward. To practice this, stick to your opponent's elbow and let him try to escape. As with the previous exercise, use leading and momentary resistance to restrict his motion. As with wrist control, try all possible ways of control. Once you can control his elbow effectively, use your coiling jing to change your control from his wrist to his elbow and vice versa.

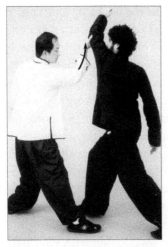 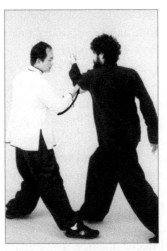

To control your opponent's elbow, lead or press it upward.

To control your opponent's elbow, you can also lead it sideways.

C. Shoulder

The shoulder is the hardest place to control, and even when you do control it, very often your opponent's hand is still alive to attack you. For this reason, controlling the shoulder is not used as often as controlling the wrist and elbow. It is hard to control the shoulder for more than a short time, so the technique is used mainly to temporarily stop the opponent's attack. Very often, it is used to enhance your control of the situation and to make your opponent lose his stability or balance.

There is no specific training for shoulder control; instead, it is used together with other techniques.

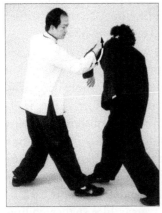 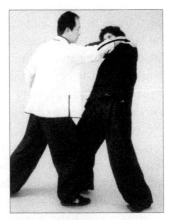 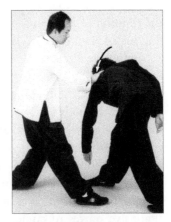

Controlling the shoulder by pushing it backward.

Controlling the shoulder by pushing it to the side.

Controlling the shoulder by pushing it downward.

Once you have attained some proficiency in the above na training, you should then practice using both hands to control one of the opponent's arms at either the wrist and elbow, or the elbow and shoulder. You should also practice using both hands to control both of your opponent's arms at either the wrists or elbows. These exercises will familiarize you with the various ways of controlling the opponent's arms and teach you to switch your control from one arm to the other as the situation changes.

However, in order to skillfully change your control from your opponent's wrist to his elbow, the elbow to the shoulder, or vice versa, you must also know two other important training exercises: coiling and sticking. Skillful hand coiling allows you to transfer from one joint to the other without a break in your sticking. Coiling and sticking are closely related and assist each other. As with a snake crawling along a tree branch, if it doesn't stick, it won't be able to coil around the branch, and if it doesn't coil, it won't be able to move forward. In the next section, we will discuss these two trainings. Remember: this is only a guideline for practice. You must keep researching with your partners for a more advanced practice.

3. Coiling and Sticking Hands Training

The purpose of sticking hands training is to practice adhering and sticking. Adhere-stick jing is one of the most basic and important jing in taijiquan practice. Without this jing, you will not be able to listen, and without listening, you will not be able to understand and react to an attack. The more you develop your sticking capability, the more your pushing hands will improve. Adhere-stick jing is the jing of not losing or separating from the opponent. This means that you should adhere-connect, stick-follow with your opponent all the time. In order to do this, first you must be so soft that you stick like glue, and you must be able to coil like a snake creeping around a tree branch. You must carefully listen and distinguish the substantial and insubstantial of your opponent, then you will be able to connect and follow. Adhere-stick training cannot be separated from the training of other jing such as coiling, drilling, and silk-reeling jing. Naturally, other jing such as neutralizing, leading, and controlling jing are also closely involved.

Before we discuss the practice of adhering and sticking, we would like to discuss coiling jing training first. There are many ways to coil in taijiquan. Two types of coiling are especially important: coiling of the hands and arms and coiling of the whole body. The coiling of the body enables you to use your waist to lead the hands for neutralizing, leading, and controlling. It also allows you to coordinate your body with your steps and helps you to accumulate jing in your chest. Here we will discuss coiling training for the hands and arms. Coiling training for the whole body will be discussed in the silk-reeling training section later. Coiling cannot be separated from adhere and stick. If one knows coiling well, he must also know adhere and stick well and vice versa. Usually, coiling is used in aggressive moves to circle your arms around the opponent's arms like snakes coiling around branches. Your hands must coil when you adhere and stick to the opponent's joints, such as his elbow or wrist, and especially when you wish to move from one joint to another. When you use coiling jing, your adhering and sticking will become alive and adaptable. Without coiling jing, your sticking and adhering will be like a dead snake wrapped around a branch.

Hand coiling jing training trains you to coil your hands and transfer your control from joint to joint. The series of figures below show the single-hand right coiling by which you transfer your hand from the opponent's wrist to his elbow. The following series of figures show the single hand left coiling and transferring.

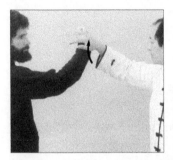 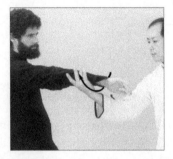 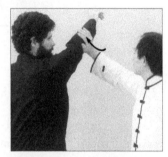

Single-hand right coiling used to transfer your hand from the opponent's wrist to his elbow.

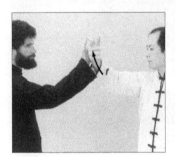 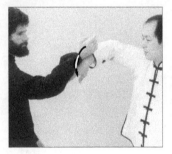 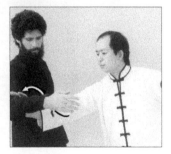

Single-hand left coiling and transferring.

Remember that the major purpose of hand coiling is to coil your hand from one joint to another on your opponent's arm so that you can control him and put him into a passive position. Therefore, once you have successfully coiled from one joint to another, you should coil your hand to a position that allows you to use sticking na effectively. Sticking na has been discussed above. However, there is another na commonly used by taijiquan martial artists—qin na. One of the categories of this na is called cavity press or nerve press. In cavity press or nerve press na, you press the opponent's cavities or nerves around the joints to numb and incapacitate the joint. The most commonly cavities used for control are neiguan (內關) (P-6) on the wrist joint, quchi (曲池) (LI-11) and xiaohai (小海) (SI-8) on the elbow joint, and the median nerve on the shoulder.

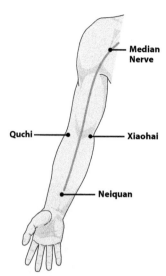

Median
Nerve

Quchi

Xiaohai

Neiquan

Common cavities used for
control.

Once you have coiled your hand to the opponent's joints, your fingers should automatically touch the above cavities or nerves in case you wish to control him.

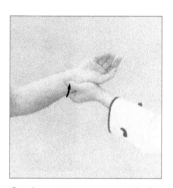
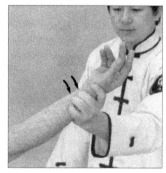

On the wrist, you can grab the cavity with your thumb or fingers.

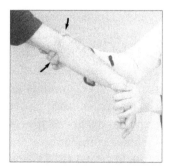
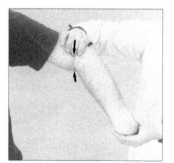

Two possible grabs on the elbow.

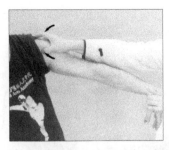 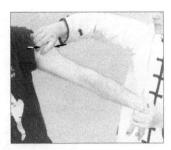

Two possible grabs on the shoulder.

To practice, start with single-hand coiling, using either hand to coil either of the opponent's arms both clockwise and counterclockwise. That means there are eight possible ways to coil. We will present here only one example; you should be able to easily figure out the other possibilities. In this example, your opponent's left leg is forward while your right leg is forward.

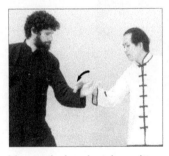 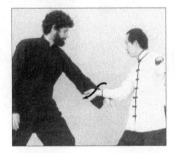

Your right hand sticks to his left wrist.

Coil your arm forward to his elbow.

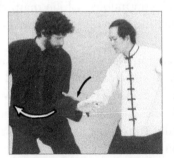 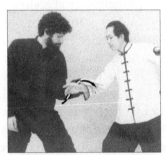

Your opponent should follow your coiling circle and twist his body to the side to escape from your control.

His hand should stick to your wrist and coil toward your elbow the same as you did to him. This exercise can be repeated continuously back and forth.

However, in a real situation, you commonly use both hands to do the job, which makes your control of him through his arm more secure.

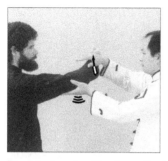 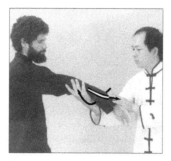 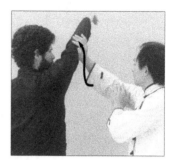

Double-hand coiling from the inside.

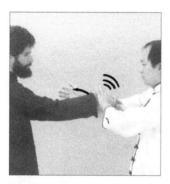 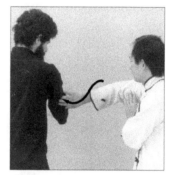

Double-hand coiling from the outside.

You can practice double-hand coiling in a continuous fashion many different ways: coiling up and down your partner's arm, switching from arm to arm, and eventually also stepping back and forth as well as sideward.

In a real fight, when your opponent is coiling around your arm for an attack, you have two options. First, you can skillfully rotate and circle your elbow and arm to reverse the situation as you would do if he were using na on your wrist and elbow. For example, if your opponent uses both hands to control your wrist and elbow, drop your elbow and coil clockwise to reverse the situation. Naturally, the coiling of your hands and arms must always be coordinated with the coiling of your whole body so that you move as a unified whole. The other way to deal with the opponent's coiling is to stick and follow, leading his arms into a disadvantageous situation. You should understand that it is easy to stick when you coil forward. However, when you coil backward you can lose contact with your opponent very easily unless you know how to adhere-connect and stick-follow well. Therefore, we will discuss sticking and leading training.

There are two occasions when you need to stick and lead. The first occasion is when your opponent is attacking you with either a strike or push, or coiling in to control you. The other occasion is when your attack is being led away and your opponent takes the opportunity to attack. You must stick to his attack and lead it into emptiness.

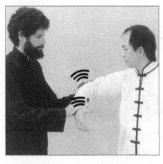

Your opponent uses both hands to control your wrist and elbow.

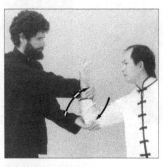

Drop your elbow.

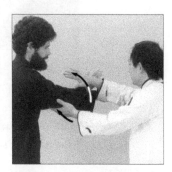

Coil clockwise to reverse the situation.

Because sticking and leading techniques are alive and vary according to the actual situation, it is hard to devise rules or routine practice. If you understand the theory and principles thoroughly, you can work at applying them in the various pushing-hands exercises. We will present here only two typical examples in hopes that they stimulate you to discover other examples.

The first example is coiling, leading, and attacking.

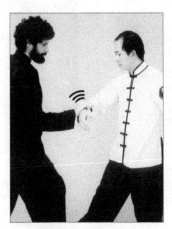

Your partner pushes your wrist with his hand.

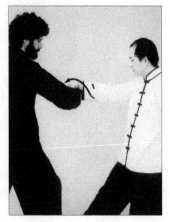

As he pushes, coil your hand around his pushing arm.

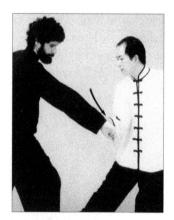

Lead it to the side.

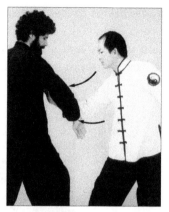

You can take this opportunity to attack. Naturally, your opponent can stick and lead your hand to the side to avoid your attack. You neutralize and attack again.

The second example is to stick and lead the opponent's forward coiling aside.

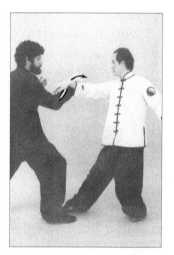

Your opponent uses his right hand to coil forward clockwise around your right arm.

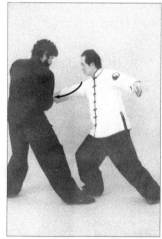

Lead him to the side with your right arm.

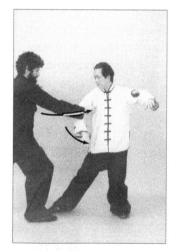

He will then immediately attack your chest with his fist. Follow his attack, stick, and lead it to the side.

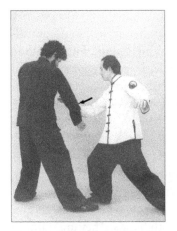
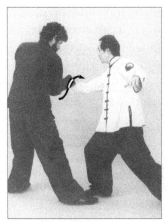
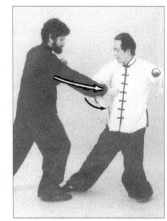

Your partner can counter by coiling counterclockwise and then attacking.

You can stick and lead his hand to your left, leading his coiling into emptiness.

In a real fight you would most probably use both of your hands to stick and lead. You can change from single to double or from opposite to same side, and you should mix forward and backward coiling. If you stick and lead skillfully, then you can trick your opponent into thinking that you are coiling in with your right hand when in fact you are really entering from your left side. Substantial and insubstantial should be exchanged to mystify your opponent. This training will greatly improve your listening, understanding, neutralizing, coiling, yielding, and leading, and give you a firm foundation for pushing hands.

Even if you do not have a partner, you can still practice your coiling, sticking, and leading by yourself.

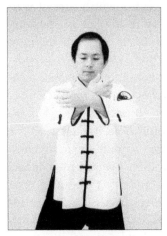
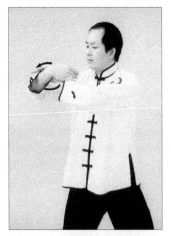
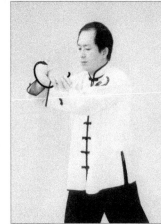

Cross your forearms in front of your chest.

Use one hand to coil around the other and lead it. Go back and forth, experimenting with different ways of coiling and controlling.

After you have mastered coiling and adhering-sticking training, you should practice using these jing in coordination with other jing such as neutralizing, leading, controlling, and drilling jing. This will lead you to the door to pushing hands. Furthermore, after you complete the training in this chapter, experiment with mixing and adapting the techniques so that they are alive. Remember that this book can only give you an introduction and guidelines. You must ponder, practice, and create to understand the subject thoroughly.

4. Jing Balance Training

Balance training includes posture, yi, and qi balance, and finally the mixture of the three. Once you understand balance, you have caught the trick to jing and have entered the door to the secrets of taijiquan. You may have seen taijiquan practitioners standing in the mountain-climbing stance pushing a wall or tree with both hands. They are training jing balance. Remember the verse from Chang, San-Feng's *Taijiquan Classic*: "If there is a top, there is a bottom; if there is a front, there is a back; if there is a left, there is a right." That means that if you intend to push a car forward, you must push your rear foot backward first. In order to generate strong forward jing, your yi must concentrate on the rear first. Once you coordinate this yi and qi to support the posture's jerking motion, you will be able to make the jing reach its maximum.

To train jing balance, stand in the mountain-climbing stance and have your partner push your forearm with both hands. This lets both of you train, so both of you should concentrate your yi and balance your forward arm or hands with the rear foot. The muscles should be as relaxed as possible. In the beginning, your muscles will naturally take the main role in pushing and resisting. However, when you have developed your yi and qi over a long time, they will take over control, and your muscles will be less important. After you have trained for a long time and have significantly cut down the use of your muscles, have your partner push you with quick jing and try to bounce his pushing jing backward to him. This is how to train the ability of borrowing jing.

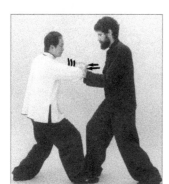

Jing balance training.

To develop balance in your offensive jing, practice techniques on a bag, wall, or partner. For example, you can practice wardoff with your forearm on your partner's chest. To avoid injury, your partner should hold his arms on his chest. In the beginning, apply your wardoff jing to his chest slowly, emphasizing forward and backward jing balance. Gradually increase your speed and try to bounce your opponent away. For more detailed discussion and training methods, refer to the book *Tai Chi Chuan Martial Power*, 3rd edition, from YMAA Publication Center.

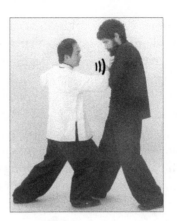

Jing offensive balance training using wardoff.

Pushing-Hands Training

1. Single Pushing Hands

The most important purpose of single pushing hands is to develop your ability at circular neutralization. It teaches you to listen, understand, neutralize, and lead. Different styles practice neutralization with different-sized circles. Generally speaking, if the defending neutralization circle is too big, you will lose your center and also expose your vital zones to attack. Not only that, but in order to use the large neutralization circle effectively, you must have extremely high listening and understanding jing. You must be able to sense the opponent's intentions so that when he moves slightly, you move first. You must be skilled in inch jing, or centimeter jing, and borrowing jing, and be able to apply the jing near the opponent's body. On the other hand, it is also dangerous for a taiji pushing-hands beginner if the neutralization circle is too small and near your body. When the small circle is used for neutralization, your opponent's jing has almost reached your body before you start to neutralize, and at this time, his jing is strongest. Unless you correctly understand your opponent's intention, your opponent's jing will easily be able to reach you. In order to use this small circle for defense, not only must your listening and understanding jing be of high level, but you must also be calm, concentrated, and agile in order to apply your yielding, neutralizing, turning, and borrowing

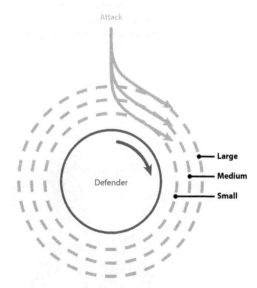

Small, medium, and large circles.

jing in a short time. Therefore, this small circle defense is not suitable for the beginner. It is best to use a medium-sized circle so that you will have enough time to sense the opponent's jing and then neutralize it. Beginners will commonly use a short resisting jing before the neutralization. This helps to sense and test the opponent's intention and also set the opponent up for your leading and controlling jing.

Practice is similar to listening and understanding training. In this exercise, as you neutralize your opponent's push, your palm turns down and continues rotating until your palm faces out. When you push, aim at your opponent's chest, not past him. When you aim your push past him, it is like punching to the side of an opponent: you will lose the sense of attack, and your opponent will not really need to neutralize your push.

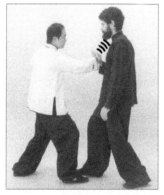

Your opponent moves forward and pushes your right forearm with his right palm.

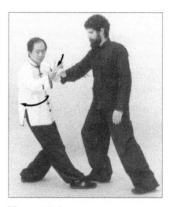

You withdraw as necessary and neutralize his push by turning your waist. Lead his attack so that it curves off to your right and his jing becomes useless.

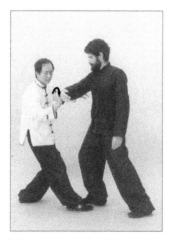

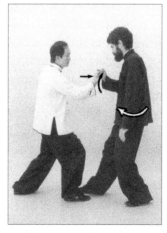

Next turn your body and palm toward him and push his forearm.

While the best neutralization with your right hand is to lead him to your right, this will frequently be unfeasible. If your partner pushes to the left side of your chest, you may not be able to lead his hand across your chest without his pushing again and reaching your body. In such circumstances, you will want to neutralize his attack to your left side, or perhaps upward or downward. You have already practiced this in the wrist neutralization training. When you lead him up or down, immediately lead his arm in a curve back to your right side and continue the exercise. When you have neutralized his attack to your left, do not then move your body forward into his arm. Instead, stay on your rear leg and turn your body to lead his arm back to your right side, and then move forward with your push.

When you practice, remember that your jing comes from your legs and is controlled by your waist. Without waist coordination, your jing and neutralization are not alive. The waist leads the arm. You must also coordinate your movements with your breathing, and possibly with the heng and ha sounds. This will help you to build up the habit of circulating qi, and raise your spirit of vitality in a natural way. In the beginning, practice slowly and keep your touch very light. Gradually speed up and use more pushing jing in the attack. You have to reach the level where, when your opponent moves fast, you respond fast, and when he moves slowly, you respond slowly.

An important function of this exercise is to train leading, controlling, and pushing jing. However, in order to make these jing effective, you must first train your adhere-stick jing; without this jing, you will lose contact with your opponent and will not be able to apply any of the other jing. Emphasize maintaining contact with the opponent wherever he moves, and only gradually become more aggressive when you can do this automatically.

2. Double Pushing Hands

After you have mastered single pushing-hands training, you should then practice double pushing hands. Single pushing hands teaches you the tricks of circling, adhering-sticking, neutralizing, leading, controlling, and pushing. However, single pushing hands can offer you only one side of the exercise. Double pushing hands is more practical and realistic because it allows you to neutralize the opponent's push with a number of different techniques. In single pushing-hands practice, your opponent can easily use his elbow to strike you, but in double pushing hands, this is considerably more difficult. Double pushing-hands training builds the foundation of all the rest of pushing hands. Therefore, you should spend time in this practice before you advance further.

Basically, double pushing hands uses the same circles and tricks of single pushing hands, but with one addition: your other hand touches your partner's elbow. The wrist and the elbow generate most of the techniques. Single pushing hands teaches you how to control your opponent's wrist, but double pushing hands teaches you how to control your partner's wrist and elbow to limit their use and mobility. You must learn how to use controlling jing on both areas.

There are four ways to neutralize the opponent's push: two fundamental and two advanced. The most fundamental technique is right neutralization.

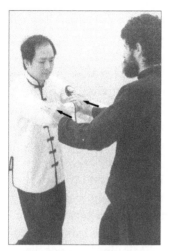

In right neutralization, when your opponent pushes your right arm, your right hand acts exactly as it did in single pushing hands.

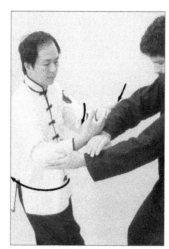

In addition, your left hand now lightly touches your partner's elbow to help lead his arm to your right, and also to prevent him from using his elbow to strike you.

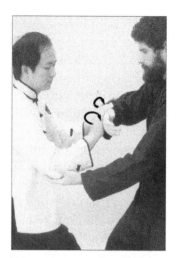

When you neutralize his push, your waist should lead your hands. After you have neutralized his push, turn your right palm to touch his wrist and slide your left hand to just below his elbow and push toward his body. Your opponent defends as you did.

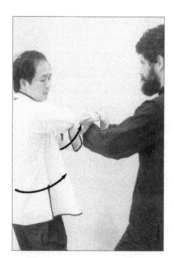

Left neutralization. Your opponent pushes your right hand toward your left. As you do this, move your left hand under your right arm and place it on the opponent's left wrist.

You may find it helpful to turn your body square toward your partner before coming forward. Beginners tend to start pushing while still turned sideways from the rollback, which causes them to push to the side of their partner. An alert partner can lead you further in that direction so that you are overextended, and then easily push you down.

The second technique is left neutralization, which is generally used when your partner attacks the upper left side of your body. In this case, as he pushes your right arm toward your left, rotate your body to the left and use your right arm to lead his jing to the left to neutralize the attack.

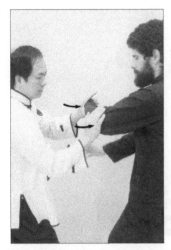
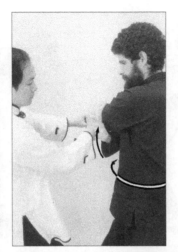
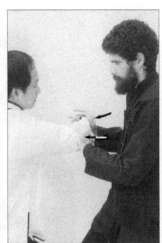

Your left hand takes over from your right hand and continues to lead his attack past you. Move your right hand to his left elbow, and when his attack is neutralized, push toward him with both hands. You are now pushing your opponent's left arm.

Your opponent can use the same technique to neutralize your push to his right. Both of you should practice the two fundamental techniques interchangeably without stopping until the exercise becomes smooth and natural.

Advanced neutralization is called mo (摸) or smearing, and is usually done when your opponent pushes your arm across your body to seal it. It is called "smearing" because your hand moves in a circular motion as if you are smearing something on a wall with your forearm. This technique relies upon the combination of adhering-sticking, coiling, and neutralizing jing.

In the next few pictures, the performer in the white shirt is doing left smearing while the performer in the black shirt is doing right smearing.

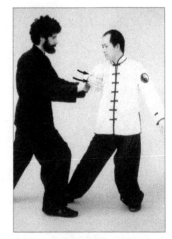

Black pushes white's forearm with both hands to the left side of white's chest.

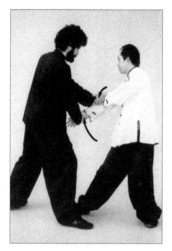 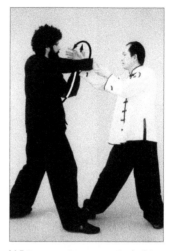

White uses his left hand to press down on black's left hand in order to control it, and at the same time circles his right arm down. While he does this, black sticks to white's right wrist with his right hand in order to prevent white from controlling his left elbow.

White continues to circle his arm counterclockwise until his right hand reaches black's elbow.

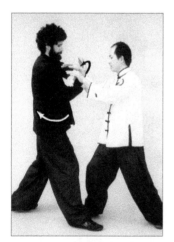 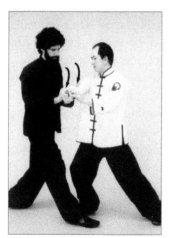 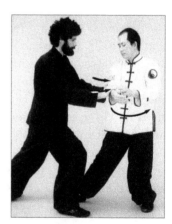

To prevent white from controlling his elbow, black pulls back his left arm and rotates his body to his right, and at the same time uses his right hand to smear away both of white's hands.

Immediately after smearing, black continues the motion and pushes white's right arm with both hands. White then twists his body to his left and repeats his counterclockwise smearing.

Smearing techniques are the foundation of the rollback jing exercises that will be discussed later. Once you have mastered your stationary double pushing-hands training, you should practice stepping into the most advantageous position for your attack. Naturally, as you step around to attack, your partner should also turn and step to avoid your attacking his open door.

After you have learned the four fundamental techniques of double pushing hands, you should learn the eight major taijiquan techniques: peng (掤) (wardoff); lu (撈) (rollback); ji (擠) (press); an (按) (push); cai (採) (pluck); lie (挒) (split); zhou (肘) (elbow stroke); kao (靠) (shoulder stroke). You must also coordinate your techniques with the five strategic movements called the five elements: jin bu (進步) (forward); tui bu (退步) (backward); zuo gu (左顧) (beware of the left); you pan (右盼) (look to the right); and zhong ding (中定) (central equilibrium). These thirteen postures form the foundation of taijiquan and lead you to hundreds of techniques.

It is not feasible to use a book to learn all the techniques derived from the thirteen postures. There are many variations for each technique, and there are further variations in how each person does particular techniques because of individual differences in understanding and experience. This chapter will teach you the fundamentals and give you guidelines so that you can research and develop on your own.

3. Wardoff

Wardoff is the technique of using your forearm to push or bounce your opponent away. It is commonly used against the chest, shoulder blade, and upper arm to cause your opponent to lose his balance and fall or be bounced away. It is especially important to use your opponent's open door when using wardoff.

A. Chest

In order to access your opponent's chest, you must first neutralize his attack and lead it to the side to expose the chest area. You must therefore know how to use coiling, neutralizing, leading, or rollback jing to do this. Naturally, you must also adjust your steps so that you can access his front open door and execute wardoff to his chest. To practice, start with your partner doing wardoff on your chest.

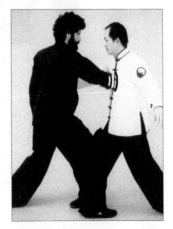

Your partner doing wardoff on your chest.

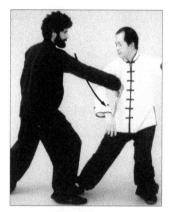

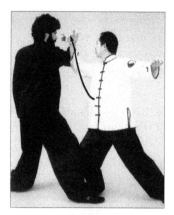

When he just begins to emit jing, yield, then turn your body to the left to neutralize his force and lead it past you. Your right arm moves forward to connect to and control his elbow or upper arm.

Immediately circle your right arm up and shift your weight to your right leg, controlling his arm and preventing further attack.

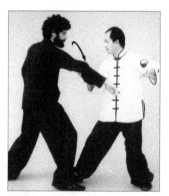

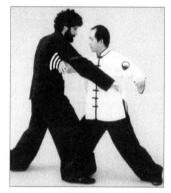

Your opponent is now in a disadvantageous position. In order to regain the advantage, he will have to push forward to neutralize your arm to his right. When this happens, follow his power and use small rollback to lead his arm away and open his chest to attack.

Finally, readjust your steps to reach his front open door and execute wardoff to his chest. For continuous practice, your partner should neutralize and counter the same way you did.

Example of a response when your opponent uses his left arm to execute wardoff to your chest.

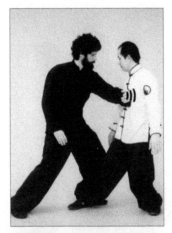

Your opponent uses his left arm to execute wardoff to your chest while your right leg is forward.

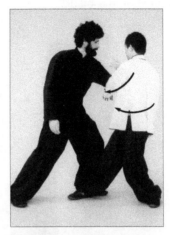

Twist your body to your right, and use your left arm to neutralize and lead his attack into emptiness.

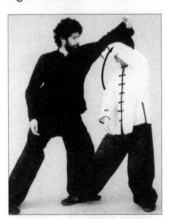

Continue to circle your left arm up to open his chest.

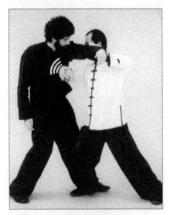

Finally, use your right arm to perform wardoff to his chest. Your partner sits back and turns to his left to repeat the same movements you have made.

B. Shoulder Blade

An example response for when your opponent uses his right arm to execute wardoff against your right shoulder blade.

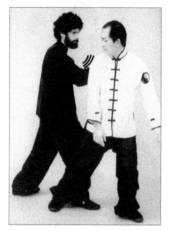

Your opponent uses his right arm to execute wardoff against your right shoulder blade.

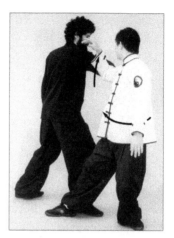

Shift your weight to your left leg, and twist your body to your right to lead his attack into emptiness.

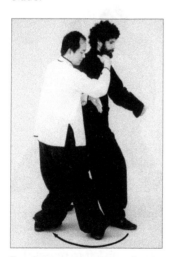

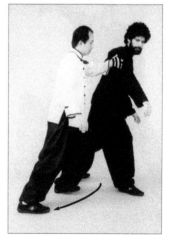

Readjust your steps so that you are behind him, and use your left arm to execute wardoff against his shoulder blade.

C. Upper Arm

When you intend to use wardoff to the opponent's upper arm, you must first neutralize his attack and lead his arm down. You can then use your forearm to perform wardoff against his upper arm. To practice, have your partner perform wardoff to your right arm with his right arm.

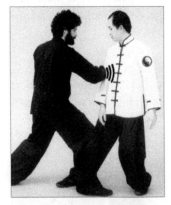

Your partner uses wardoff on your right arm with his right arm.

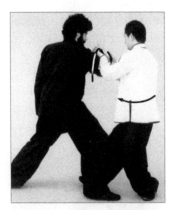

Neutralize and lead his wardoff to your right and press it down with both arms.

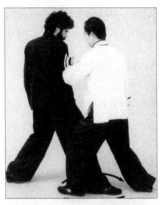

Immediately step to readjust your position and use your left leg to seal his right leg, and at the same time use your left arm to perform wardoff against his arm.

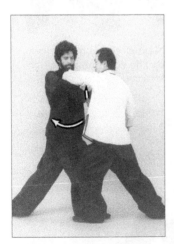

Your partner should then turn to his left and neutralize your attack with his left hand.

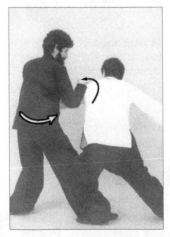

He immediately adjusts his feet so that his right leg is behind your left leg, and then presses down your upper arm with his right hand.

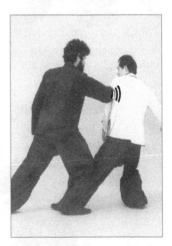

He should then immediately execute wardoff against your left arm with his right arm.

Because there are often several ways to neutralize, this exercise can have many variations. Practice using wardoff after all of the possible neutralization.

4. Rollback

Rollback is generally practiced together with press, push, or wardoff. Therefore, when you practice, eventually you are practicing the mixture of all four trigrams. This will make your pushing-hands exercise alive and closer to the practical usage. Rollback has two forms: small rollback (xiao lu, 小撮) and large rollback (da lu, 大撮).

Small Rollback

In small rollback practice, the range is shorter than in large rollback, and the footwork is usually not as important. To practice, have your partner press you with his right wrist forward.

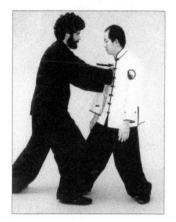
Your partner presses you with his right wrist forward.

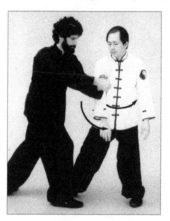
Sit back and turn your body so that your right arm leads his push to your left side.

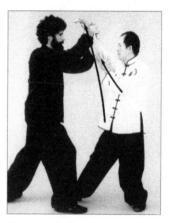
Next circle both your arms up and coil around his right forearm.

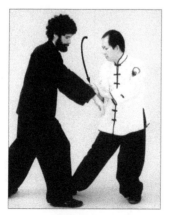
Lead it to your left side.

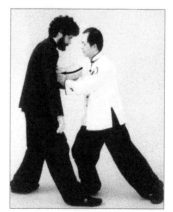
Immediately press his chest with both hands. Your partner does the same thing to you for continuous practice.

If your partner presses your right upper arm with his left wrist while his left leg forward, you can also neutralize his press to your left.

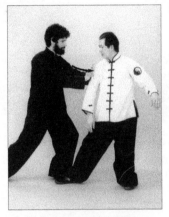

Your partner presses your right upper arm with his left wrist while his left leg is forward.

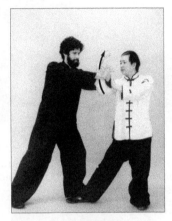

Place your right hand between both his arms, circle his arm upward, and coil around his left elbow.

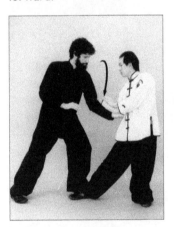

Lead it to your left.

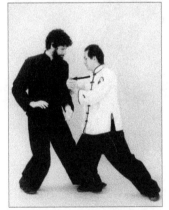

Finally, use your right wrist to press his left upper arm.

Large Rollback

In stationary large rollback practice, stand with your right leg forward while your partner stands with left leg forward and presses you with his left wrist or forearm. There are two ways of neutralizing his press. In both exercises, when you perform rollback, your left hand should grasp his left wrist, and your right hand should control his elbow or upper arm.

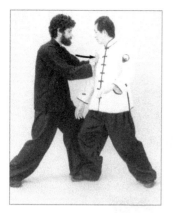 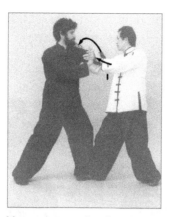 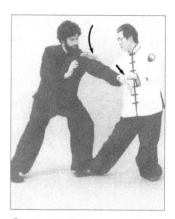

Your partner stands with left leg forward and presses you with his left wrist or forearm.

You can neutralize his press to your left with your upper arm.

Control his left arm, and then perform rollback to your left rear.

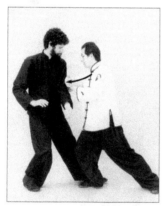 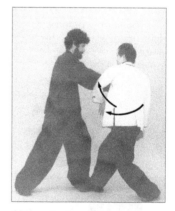

Finally, press his chest with your right wrist.

Alternatively, you can neutralize his press to your right by twisting your body and using your left upper arm.

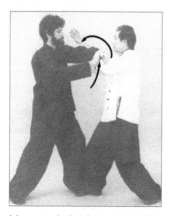 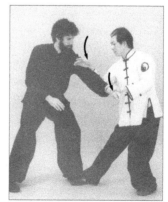

Next circle both your hands to control his left arm as you perform rollback. Finally, move forward and press.

In moving rollback training, you step back as you control his arm. When your right leg is forward and your opponent presses or pushes you with his left leg forward, you have the option of using rollback on his right or left arm. When you perform rollback against his left arm, it is the same as stationary rollback. When you perform rollback against his right arm, you have to readjust your steps so that your left leg is forward.

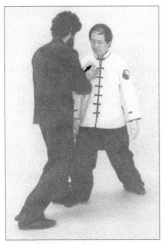

Your opponent presses you with his left leg forward.

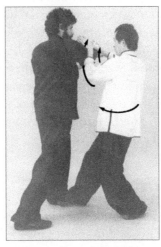

Neutralize his press to your right.

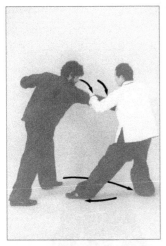

Next readjust your right leg, and at the same time circle and coil both your hands until you control his right wrist and elbow as you perform rollback.

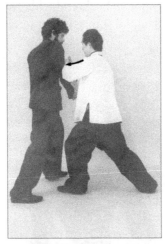

If you wish to do a continuous exercise, don't perform rollback so far that your partner falls, but instead deliver rollback partially so that your partner is off balance to the front, and as he pulls back, press him.

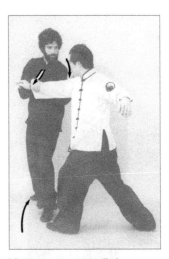

Your opponent will then readjust his legs and neutralize your press to continue the practice.

The more you practice, the better, smoother, and more continuous you will be. From this continuous practice, you learn how to set up your steps; how to connect, stick, and adhere; and how to be alive.

5. Press

Press uses the wrist or occasionally the forearm, with the support of the other hand, to apply force to the opponent to make him fall or bounce away, or sometimes to strike him. In principle, this technique is very similar to the wardoff described above; however, there are two major differences. First, because the wrist is used for press, it can reach farther than wardoff. Second, because there is support from the other hand, the jing generated can be sharper, faster, and more penetrating. It can therefore be used more effectively than wardoff for striking. The principle of setting up the legs to access the opponent's open door is the same as with wardoff. Press can also be practiced against the chest, the shoulder blade, and the upper arm.

Chest:

The exercises for practicing press on the chest are the same as the ones discussed in the section on rollback. Please refer to that section. Because the exercise of pressing the chest has been discussed in rollback, we will not repeat it here.

Shoulder Blade:

When your partner presses your right shoulder blade with his right wrist, twist your body to neutralize his press and adjust your position to reverse the situation.

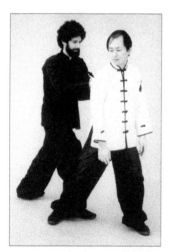
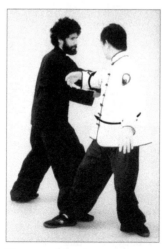
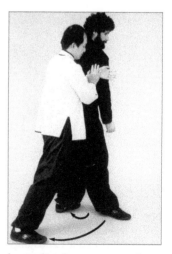

Your partner presses your shoulder blade with his right wrist.

Twist your body to your right to neutralize his press and lead it into emptiness.

Immediately step to readjust your position and use your wrist to press his shoulder blade.

To practice press as a continuous exercise, you will have to vary the target areas to maintain smoothness and continuity. In the previous instance, for example, black can turn his body to his right and press white's chest.

Upper Arm:

When your partner presses your upper arm, you can neutralize and lead his press to either your right or your left.

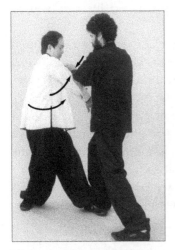 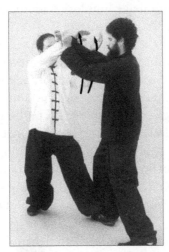 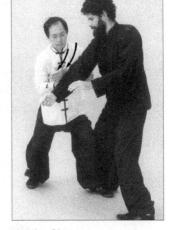

You neutralize and lead this press to your left.

Circle both of your arms to move both of his arms to your right side.

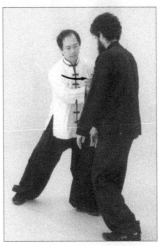

Immediately press his upper arm. When you counter his press, you should also step your left leg behind his right leg to seal his retreat or to bounce his thigh to uproot him.

6. Push

Push is similar to wardoff and press; however, there are a few differences. First, push can reach farther than wardoff and press. Second, push can be done with one or both hands. When both hands are used, they can be used for a simultaneous attack or, alternatively, one hand can set the opponent up either by controlling a joint or by pushing him off balance while the other hand delivers the actual attack. Third, when push is used for striking, it is able to do more damage than either wardoff or press. Fourth, when push is used to strike the opponent instead of bounce him away, the steps become less important because you do not have to make him lose stability. Push, as a strike, can be used anytime the opponent's vital areas are open.

Push is commonly used on the chest, arm, and shoulder blade. Sometimes it is used to push the opponent's arm down to prevent further movement. Downward push is also often used to strike the stomach area to seal the opponent's breath. In pushing-hands practice, because the striking push is dangerous, only the bouncing push is used. As a matter of fact, we have discussed single- and double-hand pushing practice when we discussed the exercises for single and double pushing hands. Once you and your partner have mastered the techniques, you should then use more jerking jing in your pushing hands so that you both get practice in both emitting and neutralizing jing.

There is another common set of two-handed pushing exercises called up and down double-hands pushing. Have your partner push your chest with both hands.

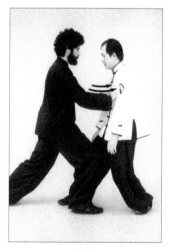 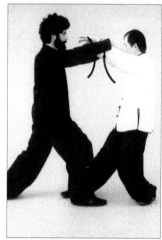

Your partner pushes your chest with both hands.

Right before his jing is emitted, neutralize his push upward with both your arms.

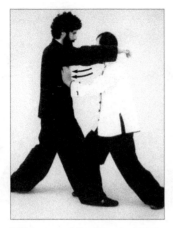 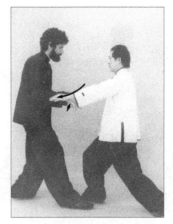

This opens his chest to your push.

Your partner neutralizes your push down and to the side and then pushes at your chest again.

7. Pluck and Rend

There are many exercises for practicing pluck and rend together. Here we will introduce four exercises as examples. There is a sideward and a downward pluck, and a forward and a sideward rend. After you have practiced these four examples, you should experiment and find additional training methods.

Strike the Tiger and Wave Hands in the Clouds

Wave hands in the clouds is used for training sideward rend. It is commonly used to rend and rotate the opponent to a disadvantageous position so that he cannot continue his attack or so that he loses his stability. To practice, have your partner grab your right wrist with his right hand, left leg forward, and punch to your head with his left hand.

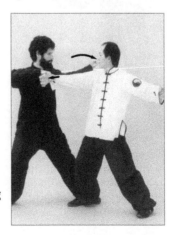

Your partner grabs your right wrist with his right hand, left leg forward, and punches to your head with his left hand.

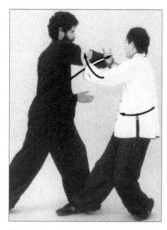 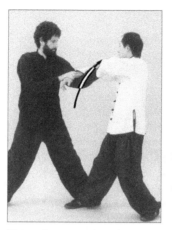 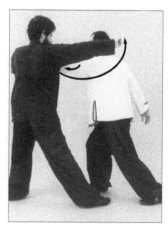

To defend against his strike, twist your body to your right while pressing his wrist with your right hand and his shoulder with your left hand.

This will prevent him from punching you with his left fist and also put him in a twisted and disadvantageous position. Your partner should then grab your left arm with his left hand and pull you to his left.

Next he steps his right leg forward and punches at your head with his right fist. You then use wave hands in the clouds to neutralize his attack and pull him to your left, and continue the exercise.

Wild Horses Shear the Mane and Wave Hands in the Clouds

This practice is similar to the last one except that your opponent attacks you with wild horses shear the mane, attempting to bounce you back with his left arm under your armpit.

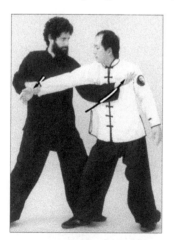 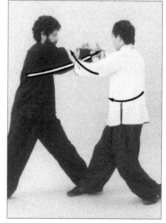

Your opponent attacks you with wild horses shear the mane, attempting to bounce you back with his left arm under your armpit.

To evade his attack, you must twist your body to your right, pressing or controlling his right wrist with your right hand and his left elbow with your left hand.

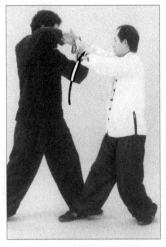 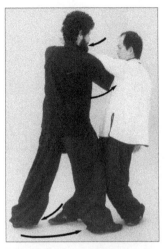

Your opponent then pulls your left wrist with his left hand.

He uses wild horses shear the mane to your left armpit area. You use pluck and rend to twist his body to the left.

Pick Up Needle from Sea Bottom and Fan Back

These two forms are first a downward pluck and then a rend upward and forward.

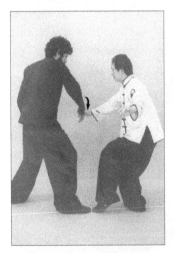 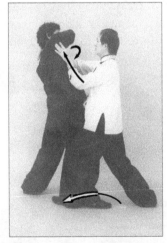 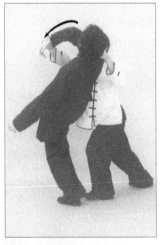

Pluck your partner's right wrist and pull it down. Your weight is on your rear foot, and only the toes of your front foot touch the floor.

Your opponent must resist your pull to avoid losing his balance. When you sense his pulling back, immediately follow his motion and step your left leg behind his right leg, and at the same time push his right wrist to his left side.

Once he has lost his balance, push him upward and to his rear, or else twist him counterclockwise to destroy his balance.

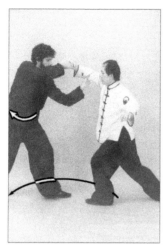

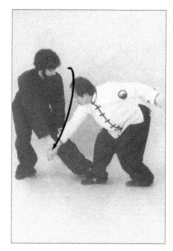

For continuous practice, when you step your left leg behind his right leg, your partner should step his right leg back and twist his body to his right to readjust his position.

As this is happening, he should also pluck your wrist and pull it down as you did to him.

Sideward Pluck and Circling Rend

This exercise is used mainly to train you in how to readjust your steps to avoid an awkward position, and also put your opponent in a disadvantageous position. These two forms are commonly used right after large rollback to make the opponent lose his balance and fall.

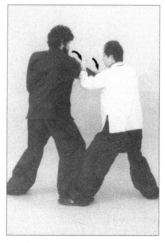

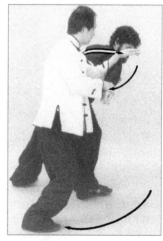

Apply large rollback to your opponent.

Step behind yourself with your rear leg, and continue to rotate your body so that your opponent loses his balance.

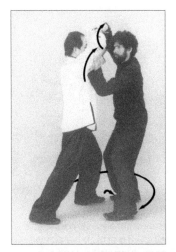
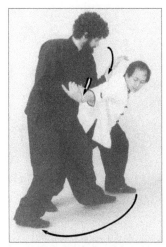

For continuous practice, when you rend your partner, he should not resist you but instead follow your pull and readjust his steps, and then pluck your arm and use circling rend on you.

8. Elbow and Shoulder Stroke

Elbow and shoulder stroke are commonly practiced with neutralization techniques such as twisting the body and plucking the wrist and elbow. In practice, these two strokes are often exchanged one for the other, depending upon your distance from your partner. The routine is therefore not rigid. To practice, you must first neutralize your opponent's stroke and set him up for your attack, and then use the appropriate attack. When you neutralize his stroke, you can twist your body, perform rollback, pluck, or even use your shoulder to neutralize. Here, we will introduce some examples of elbow stroke and shoulder stroke and hope this will guide you in your practice and research.

Elbow Stroke

Your opponent plucks and pulls your right arm forward and at the same time strikes you with his left elbow in your armpit area.

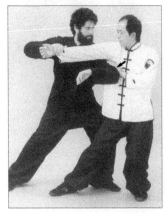

Your opponent plucks and pulls your right arm forward and at the same time strikes you with his left elbow in your armpit area. Stop his elbow attack with your left hand while sitting back to reduce the power of his attack.

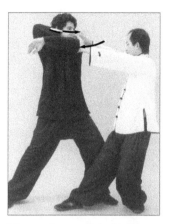 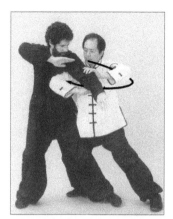

Next pull your right hand back while your left hand pushes forward to expose his left armpit area to your attack.

Immediately use your right elbow to attack his armpit area. Naturally, your opponent can do the same thing to you by first neutralizing your strike and then attacking you again.

Another example is when your opponent attacks your right armpit area with his left elbow while his right hand grasps your right wrist.

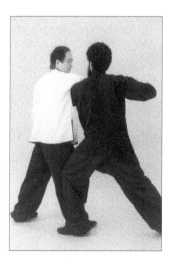 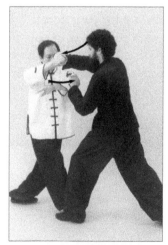

Your opponent attacks your right armpit area with his left elbow while his right hand grasps your right wrist.

You can use wave hands in clouds to pluck and turn him and twist your body to the right so that you avoid the stroke and put your opponent in a disadvantageous situation.

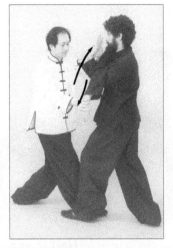

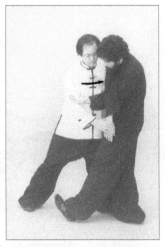

Continue to pull his right wrist to his left side and at the same time pull his left arm to his right.

Finally, step your left leg forward and use your elbow or shoulder to strike his chest.

Shoulder Stroke

Examples for when your partner uses his left shoulder to strike your chest.

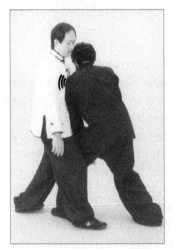

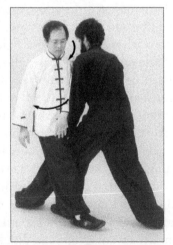

Your partner uses his left shoulder to strike your chest.

Sit back to yield, and at the same time twist your body to your right and use your left shoulder to neutralize his stroke.

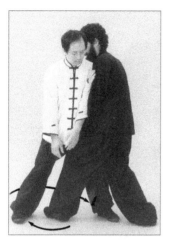 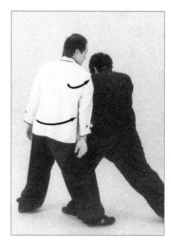 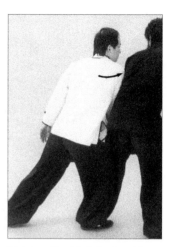

Right after your neutralization, hop to reverse your legs and strike his chest with your left shoulder. Naturally, your opponent can do the same thing to you.

Alternatively, you can neutralize his shoulder stroke to your left with your right shoulder.

Next strike his left shoulder blade with your right shoulder.

9. Silk-Reeling Training

Once you have mastered the above exercises, you will have built a firm foundation for taijiquan fighting and will have practiced stepping according to the five elements. In order for you to reach the next level of fighting skill, your steps need to automatically follow your techniques, and they must also work strategically to put the opponent in a bad situation where he is vulnerable to your attack. When the five elements are exchanged skillfully in your stepping, you will tend to move in ways that help you protect yourself, and avoid situations where the opponent has you at a disadvantage. In this five-element training, the general rule is that the stepping pattern should be circular. When your stepping is circular, you avoid channeling yourself into a corner, and you can more easily avoid using force against force. Once you have reached this level, your techniques will coordinate with your steps instead of your steps coordinating with your techniques.

In order to train this circular stepping, Chinese martial artists in internal styles use the eight trigrams (bagua, 八卦) as a pattern. This pattern shows the ways to move which are safe and unsafe, advantageous and disadvantageous. The student will practice walking around the pattern until he can naturally move correctly, with no mistakes. In internal Chinese martial arts, this training is called zou bagua (走八卦), which means walking the eight trigrams. Usually, the walking patterns of the various styles are somewhat different, depending on the style's techniques, characteristics, and fighting strategies, and each style keeps its pattern secret. Unfortunately, due to the neglect of taijiquan's martial side, taiji's bagua walking training has almost been forgotten.

In this subsection we would like to introduce one of the most basic taiji bagua walking exercises, which is combined with silk reeling. Silk-reeling training is a mixture of many basic taijiquan jing such as coiling, wrapping, drilling, neutralizing, leading, and adhering-sticking. Silk reeling doesn't train just your hands and arms, but it also trains your whole body to move coherently. Silk-reeling exercises can be practiced stationary and moving. Stationary training has been discussed in my book *Tai Chi Chuan Martial Power: Advanced Yang Style*, 3rd edition, and will not be repeated here. We will now introduce the moving silk-reeling training that follows the bagua pattern. Hopefully, this training will help you understand the foundation of the deeper taijiquan fighting art.

There are many ways to walk the bagua circle, such as right-hand clockwise circling with forward clockwise walking, right-hand clockwise circling with backward counterclockwise walking, left-hand counterclockwise circling with forward counterclockwise walking, and left-hand counterclockwise circling with backward clockwise walking. It would be impossible to discuss all the possibilities in detail. In this section we will introduce only one example—right-hand clockwise circling with forward clockwise walking. It is up to you to practice, ponder, and research, and to find the other possibilities. Remember that taijiquan training should be alive, so as long as you follow the principles, your training will be worthwhile.

In this bagua walking practice, your hands should circle according to the pattern of the stationary silk-reeling training that was discussed in the book *Tai Chi Chuan Martial Power*. The movement of your hands should coordinate with your stepping.

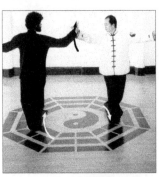 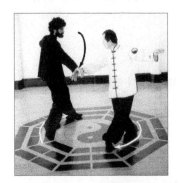 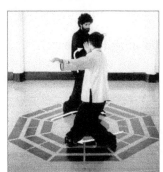

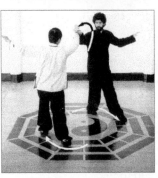 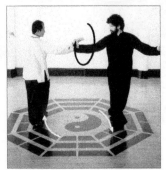 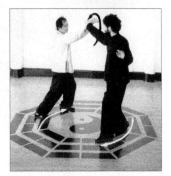

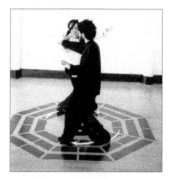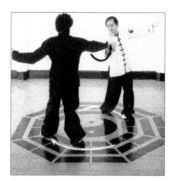

Basic taiji bagua walking exercise.

3-6. Martial Applications of Pushing Hands

There are many martial applications that can be derived from the previous fundamental pushing-hands exercises. Whether these applications are deep or shallow depends on the understanding of the individual. However, regardless of the depth of the applications, they can still be separated into the three categories discussed in the second chapter: downing the enemy, qin na control, and cavity strike. In this section, we will introduce some of the typical martial applications derived from the double pushing-hands exercises. Remember that this section can offer you only guidelines and examples; for more and deeper applications, you will have to ponder and dig for the buried treasure. In the following discussion, assume the person wearing the black shirt is your opponent and you are the one wearing the white.

Downing the Enemy

1. Right Neutralization (Opponent's Right Leg Forward)

Application 1

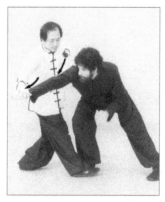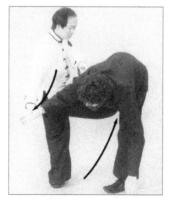

Your opponent pushes. Grasp his right wrist and pull him off balance.

At the same time, hook his right foot and sweep to the left, toppling him.

Application 2

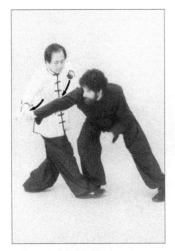 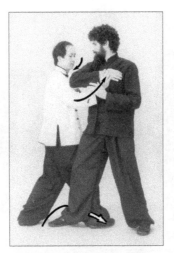 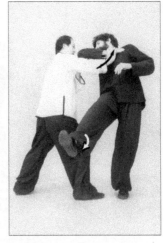

Your opponent pushes. Grasp his right wrist and pull him off balance.

If your opponent pulls back to regain his balance, step behind his right thigh and sweep the right leg backward, and simultaneously push his chest to the left to topple him.

Application 3

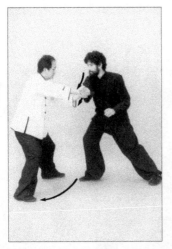 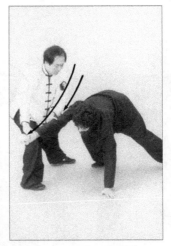

Step to the side with your right leg while locking the opponent's right arm and forcing him to the ground.

Application 4

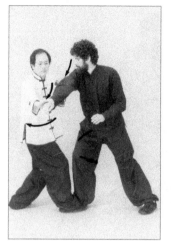 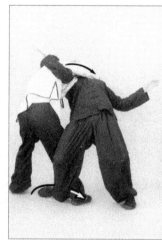

Neutralize to your right. Grasp the opponent's elbow, step your right leg behind his right foot, and lock his neck with your right arm. Sweep your right leg backward to force him to the ground.

Application 5

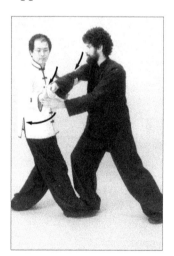 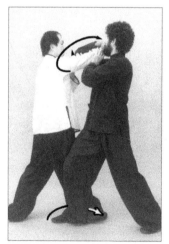 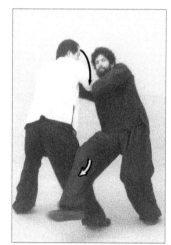

Neutralize to your right. Grasp the opponent's elbow with your left hand, and his right forearm with your right hand. Using his elbow as a pivot, bend the arm backward. Simultaneously step your right leg behind his right leg, sweeping backward and forcing him to the floor.

2. Right Neutralization (Opponent's Left Leg Forward)

Application 1

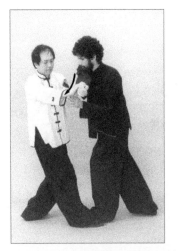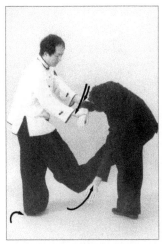

Your opponent pushes. Neutralize the force to the right. Hop forward and lock and sweep his left leg with your right leg, while at the same time pulling his right hand down.

Application 2

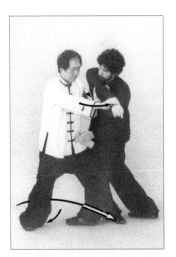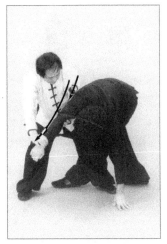

Your opponent pushes. Neutralize the power to the right, and at the same time step behind his left leg with your left leg. Sweep his left leg and pull his right hand down to make him fall.

3. Left Neutralization (Opponent's Right Leg Forward)

Application 1

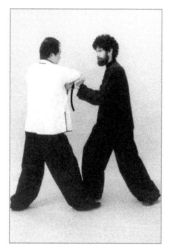 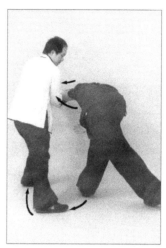

Your opponent pushes. Neutralize the opponent's push to your left. Step to the left with your left foot, pulling him off balance to his right.

Application 2

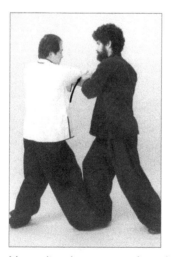 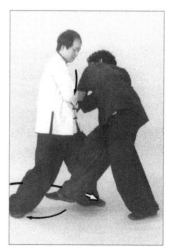

Neutralize the opponent's push to your left. Step your left leg behind his right leg and push his shoulder to topple him.

Application 3

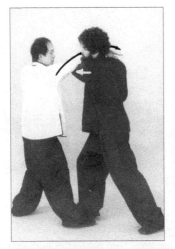 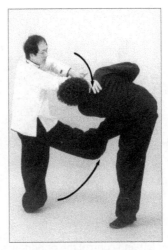

Neutralize the opponent's push to your left. Grasp the opponent's left wrist with your left hand. With your right arm, sweep his head to the right while your right leg sweeps his right leg to the left.

4. Left Neutralization (Opponent's Left Leg Forward)

Application 1

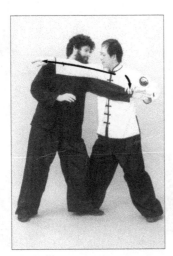 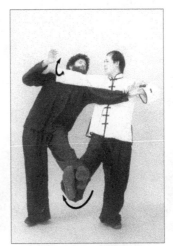

Lead your opponent's left arm out with your left hand. Step behind him, sweeping right with your right arm and left with your right leg.

Application 2

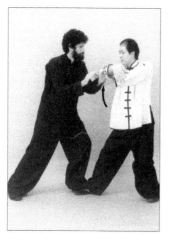 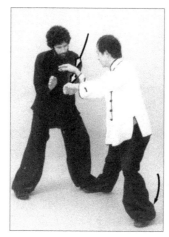 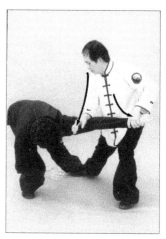

Neutralize to your left and control the opponent's left arm. Step to the left with your left leg to force him to the floor. If necessary, you can sweep his left leg with your right leg to make him fall more easily.

Qin Na Control

1. Qin Na Control of the Wrist

Application 1

Right neutralization. The opponent pushes your right arm with both hands.

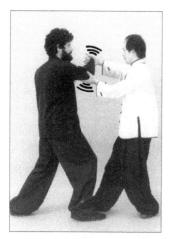 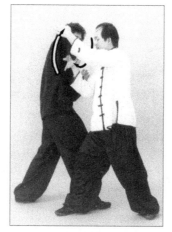 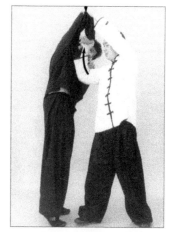

Turn to the right to neutralize the push and grasp his right wrist and elbow.	Step behind his right foot, and at the same time bend the right hand toward the wrist and move the forearm to vertical, using the elbow as the pivot.	Bend his wrist further and lift, forcing him onto his toes. Control is asserted by pushing down on the elbow and up on the hand. Applying pressure closer to the fingers results in more pain.

Application 2

Left neutralization. The opponent pushes your left arm with both hands.

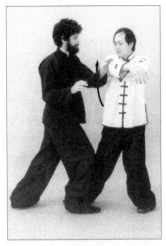 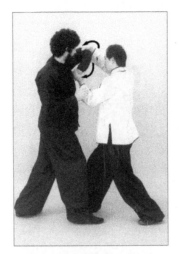 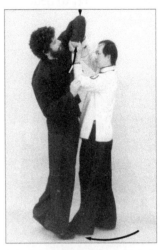

Turn to the left to neutralize the push and grasp the opponent's left wrist and elbow.

Bend the left hand toward the wrist and move the forearm to vertical, using the elbow as the pivot.

Step forward with your left foot and at the same time bend his wrist further and lift, forcing him onto his toes.

2. Qin Na Control of the Elbow

Application 1

Right Neutralization. The opponent pushes your right arm with both hands.

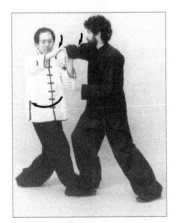 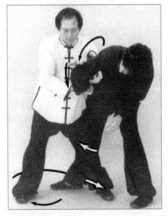 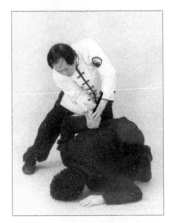

Turn to the right to neutralize the push and grasp his right wrist and elbow.

Maintain the grip on his wrist and elbow as you step your left leg forward to block his right leg.

Force him to the ground by pushing forward on his elbow while immobilizing his hand and sliding your left leg back to uproot his right leg.

Application 2

Left Neutralization. When the opponent pushes your right arm with both hands, turn to the left to neutralize the attack.

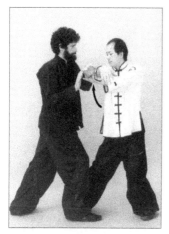 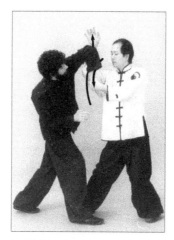 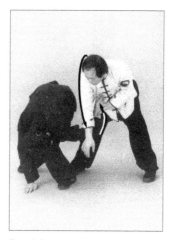

Slide his left hand to your left with your left hand, and grasp his left wrist and elbow.

Pull his wrist down and raise his elbow to unbalance him.

Bend forward, applying pressure with your right wrist to force him to the floor.

Application 3

Right Neutralization. The opponent pushes your right arm with both hands.

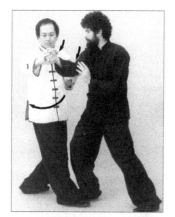 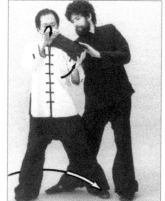 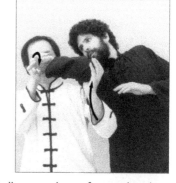

Turn to the right to neutralize the push and grasp his right wrist and elbow.

Maintain the grip on wrist and elbow, and step forward with your left leg. While keeping his arm bent, turn your body to the right and lift his elbow above his wrist and shoulder, and at the same time twist his hand outward. This movement may be difficult to understand at first but is well worth learning because it is so simple to apply when you understand it.

Application 4

Left Neutralization. When your opponent pushes your right arm with both hands, turn to the left to neutralize the push.

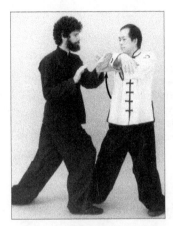 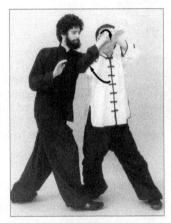 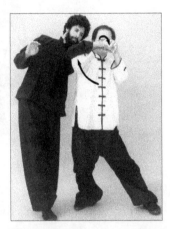

Use your left hand to lead his left arm to your left.

Grasp his left wrist with your left hand and hook his elbow with your right wrist. Pivot further to the left while sliding your right hand up to grasp his wrist, and twist his hand toward himself.

Raise your right arm to lift his elbow and force him onto his toes.

3. Qin Na Control of the Shoulder

Application 1

Right Neutralization. The opponent pushes your right arm with both hands.

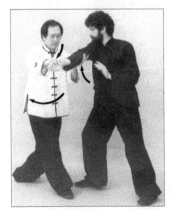

Turn to the right to neutralize the push and grasp his right wrist and elbow. Maintain the grip on his wrist and elbow, and step your left leg in to block his right leg.

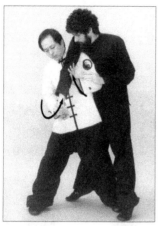

Push your left shoulder into his right armpit, and simultaneously lift up with your shoulder and push his wrist toward your shoulder. Keep his arm straight as you push to force him to his toes.

Application 2

Left Neutralization. The opponent pushes your left arm with both hands.

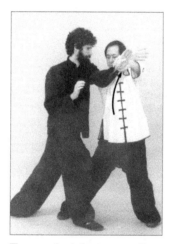

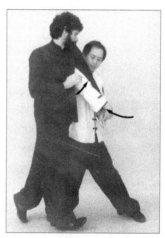

Turn to the left to neutralize the push. Grasp his left wrist with your left hand, and press in his elbow with your right forearm.

Push your right shoulder into his left armpit, and simultaneously lift up with your shoulder and push his wrist toward your shoulder, keeping his arm locked to force him to his toes. Pressure can also be generated by pushing against his elbow with your right hand.

4. Qin Na Control of the Neck

Application 1

Right Neutralization. The opponent pushes your right arm with both hands.

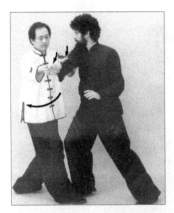 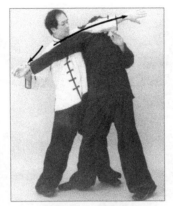 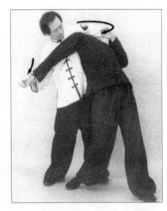

Turn to the right to neutralize the push. Grasp his right wrist and elbow.

Maintain the grip on his wrist, and step behind his right leg with your left leg and thrust your left arm over his arm to catch his neck.

To lock his neck and control him, wrap your arm around his neck and turn your trunk to the left.

Application 2

Left Neutralization. The opponent pushes your left arm with both hands.

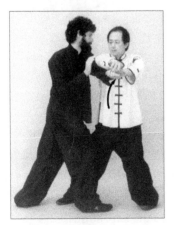 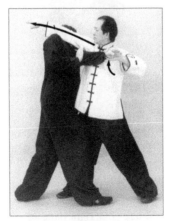 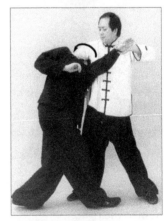

Turn to the left to neutralize the push. Grasp his left wrist with your left hand, and control his elbow with your forearm.

Maintain the grip on his wrist, and thrust your right arm over his arm to catch his neck.

Crook your right arm downward as you turn your trunk to the right, locking his neck and controlling him.

Cavity Strike

1. Right Side

Application 1

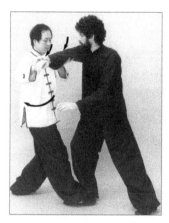 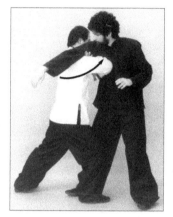

Neutralize the opponent's push to the right.

Step your right leg forward and strike his upper right chest with your right elbow to seal the breath.

Application 2

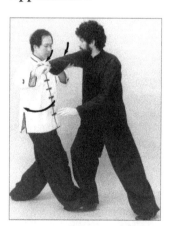 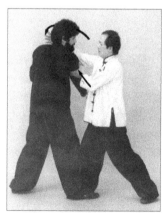 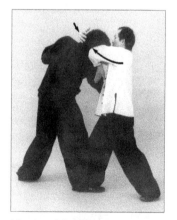

Neutralize the opponent's push to the right.

Step your right leg forward and use your right hand to grab his head.

Next pull his head down and to the left and strike his temple with the point of your elbow.

Application 3

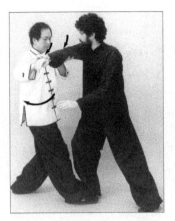 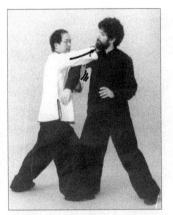

Neutralize the opponent's push to the right.

Reach over his arm and file strike the side of his neck with the edge of your hand to seal the vein. This technique will seal the oxygen supply to the brain and cause unconsciousness.

Application 4

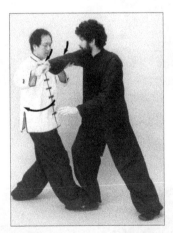 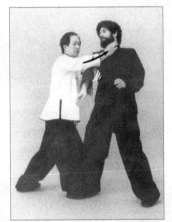

Neutralize the opponent's push to the right.

Use your right hand to reach over his arm and grasp his windpipe to seal the breath. If you squeeze until your fingers meet behind the windpipe you will displace the bone in the throat and cut off his breath. This move is usually fatal.

Application 5

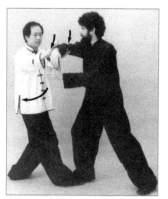

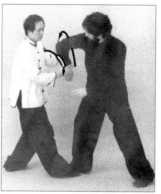

Neutralize the opponent's push. Direct his right arm down.

You then have a number of options for your strike, including cavity strike to the armpit.

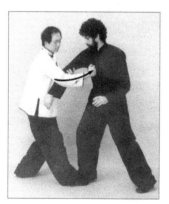

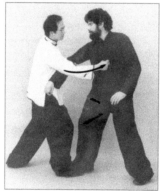

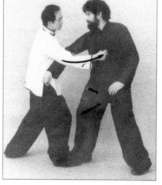

You could also cavity strike to the upper nipple to seal the breath.

Or you could cavity strike to the solar plexus.

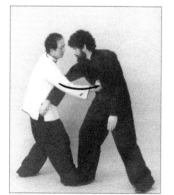

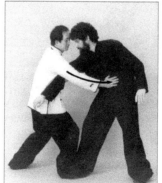

Or you could cavity strike to the liver.

2. Left Side

Application 1

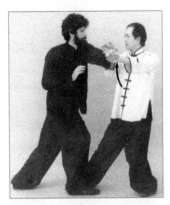 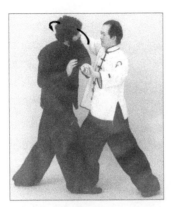 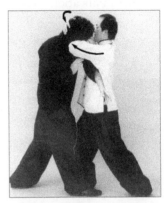

Neutralize the opponent's push to the left.

Grab the back of his head with your right hand.

Strike the bridge of the nose or the temple with your left elbow.

Application 2

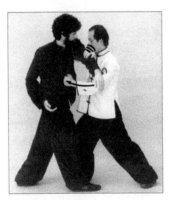 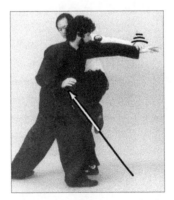

Neutralize the opponent's push. Use your left hand to strike his spleen.

Or use your left knee to kick the groin.

As mentioned, it is impossible to include all the martial applications that can be derived from pushing-hands practice. What you should learn and understand is the principle of the applications, for this will help you to learn to analyze the techniques and also to discover for yourself how to take advantage of whatever situation you find yourself in. In this case, you will have learned the trick of making a rock into a piece of gold, and you will have a chance to become a real master.

Reference

Tai Chi Theory and Martial Power: Advanced Yang Style, 3rd edition, Appendix A, by YMAA Publication Center.

Chapter 4: Analysis of the Taiji Fighting Set

4-1. Introduction

Many taijiquan practitioners misunderstand the taiji fighting set and treat it as something that should not be attempted until their skill is at a very high level. As a matter of fact, the practice would benefit midlevel students, as long as they take extra care not to build up bad habits. The fighting set is a combination of techniques from pushing hands and the solo sequence, and serves as a bridge connecting pushing hands with real fighting. Like pushing hands, it teaches you how to sense your opponent's actions and intentions, but it also teaches footwork and how to set up your strategy, knowledge necessary for a more realistic and alive practice. Anyone who is good at the solo sequence and pushing hands should be able to easily learn the fighting set and make it part of his practice routine. When doing the fighting set, you must still follow all the basic principles that were emphasized in pushing hands, such as differentiating substantial and insubstantial, not meeting force with force, and always adhering to the opponent. Once you have learned the fighting set, you must learn how to analyze it so that you understand not just how to do a particular technique but also why. You must understand the set well enough so that it becomes alive. Then you can be creative and vary the way you practice.

This set can only offer you guidelines for taijiquan fighting. In a real fight, you will generally need more techniques and skills than what you have practiced in pushing hands and the fighting set. Most external Chinese styles have more than one fighting set so that students can prepare for a greater number of the situations that occur in real fights. Also, most masters of external styles encourage qualified students to create fighting sets for practice. This forces them to really analyze their art, and improves their free fighting. It is also desirable to do this in taijiquan once you have achieved a high level of ability and thoroughly understand the theory and techniques. If you are not qualified and you start to create, you will tend to create routines that build up bad habits, and this may get you hurt in a fight. You usually need twenty years of learning and practice before you are qualified to create a new sequence.

In this chapter we will first list and discuss the general rules that a taiji fighting set follows. We will then analyze the forms and techniques, and discuss some application options. This should help you to catch the knack of how taijiquan forms are actually used, and to learn the general rules of fighting.

4-2. General Rules and Principles

As mentioned before, every martial style has rules and characteristics that are followed in the training. If you disobey these rules, you are doing something different, not the original style. For example, Tiger style (Hu Zhua, 虎抓) specializes in using the muscles with the support of qi (hard jing) (ying jing, 硬勁). If you start following the principle of using soft against hard in your training, you are changing a basic characteristic of the style and can no longer call what you are doing Tiger style.

In Chinese martial arts, the rules and special training of each style are usually hidden in secret key words called kou jue (口訣) (oral secrets). They are also commonly hidden in poetry and songs that are secretly passed down from generation to generation. Fifteen of the taijiquan poems and songs have been included, with commentary, in the appendix of the book *Tai Chi Chuan Martial Power*, from YMAA Publication Center. When you practice, if you do not follow the rules and principles originally stated in these songs, you are doing something else that cannot be called taijiquan.

In Chinese martial arts, there are also many general rules and principles that must be obeyed, regardless of which style you are in. For example, the principle of the open door and the general rules for protecting the open door are valid for all styles, because they are the rules of fighting. Any style that does not obey these rules and principles is a bad style.

Taijiquan has many rules and principles of its own. As you train, you may tend to emphasize particular aspects of the art, or devise training methods that develop particular skills. This is how the various styles of taijiquan originated. Over the years, each style has developed its own secret songs and poems that express and define its character. However, all taijiquan styles must still follow the basic classical poetry, or else they will stray from the true nature of taijiquan.

We will now list the general rules and principles of taijiquan. If you follow them conscientiously, you will learn taijiquan with a minimum of error and may someday be able to create your own sequence.

Rules and Principles

1. Soft against Hard

The first and most important principle of taijiquan is soft against hard. If you disobey this principle, you are in conflict with the original idea of taijiquan. In order to train using weakness against strength, you must thoroughly understand yielding, neutralizing, and leading. Soft against hard means sticking and following, and not resisting. If you resist, then what you are doing is more like an external style. Of course, there are times when you are obliged to resist, but your resistance should be of a very short duration. You use it only when you must borrow some time to escape from a very disadvantageous situation.

2. Slow Follows Slow and Fast Follows Fast

This is probably the second most important principle in taijiquan. Slow follows slow and fast follows fast means adhere-stick. When you adhere-stick skillfully, your opponent feels that you are like a piece of flypaper sticking to him and he cannot get rid of you. This is the technique of "not losing your opponent." If you can use adhere-stick well, together with yielding, neutralizing, and leading, you will be able to put your enemy in a passive and disadvantageous situation. In order to adhere-stick, you must be good at listening and understanding. All of these are the roots of taijiquan. Without these roots, your taijiquan will be dead.

3. Access Open Doors and Windows

Martial artists in every style need to know how to access the opponent's open doors and how to open his windows. You must know your opponent's open doors, whatever stance he uses, and you must also know where your own open doors are so that you can prepare for your opponent's attack. A fighting set must train both sides to access and defend the open doors, which helps both sides to develop a sense of enemy. You must also know how to open the windows whenever the opponent's doors are closed or when he is prepared. The techniques that taijiquan uses are very different from most external styles. Taijiquan specializes in using coiling, silk reeling, wrapping, and controlling to open the opponent's window for an attack. In accessing the open door and in opening the windows, footwork is extremely important. If you do not understand the trick of using your footwork to set up fighting strategy, your opponent will not have to worry too much about his doors and windows and will be able to seal them tightly, rendering your techniques ineffective.

4. Jing Has Root

Sometimes people create fighting sets with techniques that would not be able to hurt the enemy if they were used in a real fight. This is because their fighting set does not follow the principle of rooting the jing. Every jing needs a root in order to generate power, just like an arrow needs a bow to accumulate and emit energy. The root of jing can be in the legs, waist, shoulder, chest, or even the elbow. If you create a fighting set with techniques that have no power, then even if you can access the enemy's vital areas, you will not be able to attack them effectively. Furthermore, such techniques will only create opportunities for your opponent to attack you. Therefore, in every technique, you should be able to generate jing quickly and effectively so that you will be able to use it in a real fight. In addition to having a root to the jing, each technique must also be able to direct the jing to the target easily. If this cannot be done, the jing is useless. Therefore, you must consider the root of jing as well as the places that coordinate and direct it—the waist and elbows.

5. Connected and Not Broken

The techniques in a fighting set must be connected and not broken. This helps the practitioner develop a sense of realism in his give and take with his partner, and builds the habit of connecting offense and defense. For example, when you block down, you must sense that your upper body is exposed to attack. In the same way, when your opponent blocks your attack down, you should realize that his upper body is exposed and attack him immediately. This practice will help you to build up a natural sense for the connection between offense and defense. You should also understand that many techniques that are effective in a real fight are not suitable for a fighting set. An effective technique will usually put the opponent in a position where he has no defense. However, techniques like these stop the motion or disturb the continuity of a two-person set. For this reason, fighting sets tend to emphasize strategic techniques that allow both sides to practice accessing open doors and opening windows, as well as closing open doors and windows.

6. Techniques Must Be Alive and Fluid

This is related to rule 5 above. The techniques for both sides of a fighting set must be fluid and alive, or you will not be able to practice it without stopping. For example, muscular grabbing techniques should not be included, because if one side is grabbed tightly, the other side must resist and use force to escape, which would tend to stop the practice. However, it would be all right to include a grabbing technique that the other side could neutralize before complete control was gained, because it would not break the flow of the action. The set should train you to exchange substantial and insubstantial as you move smoothly from offense to defense and back.

7. Techniques Must Be Practical

When you combine techniques into a fighting set, you must understand how different situations can be advantageous or disadvantageous in a fight. If there is an awkward position, stance, or posture in the set, you will build up bad habits that will allow your opponent to attack you. For example, when your right leg is forward, your right hand will naturally become the master attacking and defending tool, and the left hand will become the assistant. This is because when your right leg is forward, your right hand is closer to your opponent than your left hand and can therefore attack and defend sooner.

In conclusion, a fighting set must obey the original rules and principles, and above all, they must make sense. The closer a set is to a real fight, the better it is. Imagination is important, but you should not lose the sense of realism. Remember that you should only create new sequences when you thoroughly understand the theory and principles of your system.

4-3. Analysis of the Taiji Fighting Set

In this section we will present the Yang-style fighting set. Remember: the most important thing this book can do for you is to start you analyzing the techniques. Until you understand why a technique is done and why it works, you will remain at the lowest level of achievement. In this section we will first describe the movements of each form and then analyze the movement and strategy. Additional possible martial applications will be discussed, but you should understand that there are so many ways to use each technique that it is impossible to discuss them all in one book. We will only introduce some obvious and typical applications. It is up to you to research and analyze the movements and discover more of the possible applications. A list of Chinese names, pronunciations, and English translations will be included in the appendix for your reference.

Note: In this chapter, the pictures that show alternate applications of the techniques that are not actually performed in the sequence will be indicated by a large dot in the upper left corner.

---

1. Step Forward for Punch (Shang Bu Chui, 上步捶)

Movements:

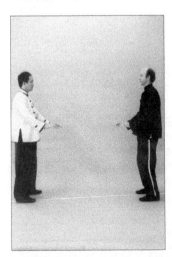 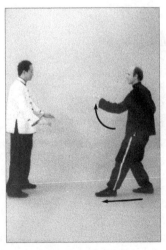 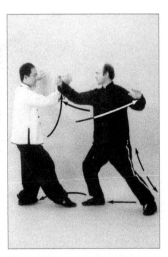

White and black stand about three steps apart with both hands in front of their waists. Black steps forward with his left leg, and then steps forward with his right leg and at the same time punches with his right hand at white's solar plexus.

Analysis:

In order to punch white's chest, black first takes two steps forward. When he punches, he uses his forward momentum along with his rooted rear leg to generate jing. In order to prevent white from using this forward momentum, he should not use all of his jing in the punch. He must hold part of the jing back so that he does not throw his body forward. Because part of the jing is withheld, the punch will not be too fast or powerful. In fact, this punch is a fake and insubstantial and is used to trick the opponent into blocking so that black can connect with his arm.

Other Options:

Because this strike is only a fake, black has already prepared for a real attack. The real attack depends on how white reacts to the fake. Remember that even though it is a fake, the attack must look powerful and real. You must force your opponent to react to it even though he knows it might be a fake.

2. Raise Hands to the Up Posture (Ti Shou Shang Shi, 提手上勢)

Movements:

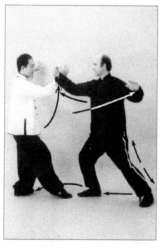

White steps his left leg backward and changes his stance into the false stance. At the same time, he raises his right hand to lead the punch up and sideward.

Analysis:

Because white does not know whether this is a real punch, he must play it safe. He steps his left leg back to yield and raises his right hand to lead the punch to his side and up. Furthermore, he also changes his stance into the false stance. This allows him to kick whenever necessary. Because of white's reaction, black must be aware of white's right leg, as his groin and dan tian are exposed to this kick.

Other Options:

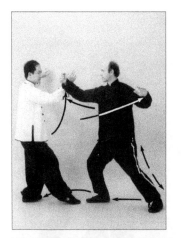 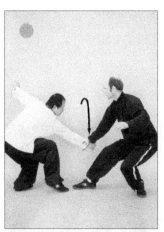

When black sees white's reaction, he can use his right hand to pluck white's right arm down. This upsets white's balance and prevents him from kicking.

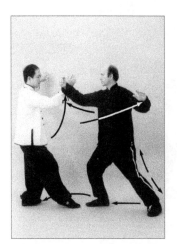 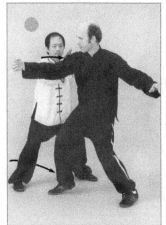 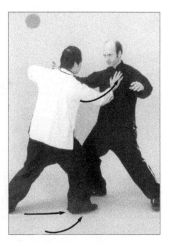

When black punches with his right hand while his right leg is forward, he has opened his doors. White can access black's right waist or shoulder blade through his right open door or his face, chest, or groin through his left open door.

3. Step Forward, Intercept, and Punch (Shang Bu Lan Chui, 上步攔捶)

Movements:

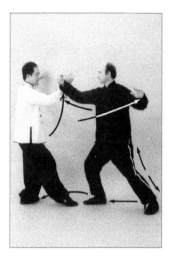 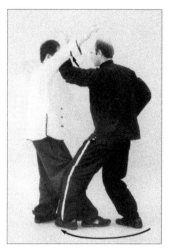

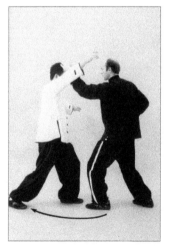 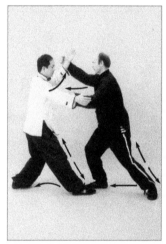

Black steps forward with his left leg and places it behind white's right leg to block his withdrawal, and at the same time lifts white's right arm to the side. White steps his right leg back to avoid having it sealed. Black steps forward with his right leg and at the same time punches with his right hand to white's chest. When this happens, white steps his left leg back and uses his left hand to deflect black's punch.

Analysis:

When black finds his right punch is blocked, he must be aware that the opponent has set his right leg up for kicking. In order to avoid this kick, he turns his body to the right and steps forward from the side, using his left leg to seal white's leg. At the same time, he moves white's right arm with his left hand to open him up to attack. White withdraws his right leg to avoid black's attempt to seal it. Black continues his attack by stepping forward with his right leg and punches white's chest. Naturally, white steps back again to keep a safe distance from black. In a fight, sense of distance is very important. If you are skillful enough to maintain the proper distance, you will be able to keep yourself safe and your opponent in a passive situation all the time.

Other Options:

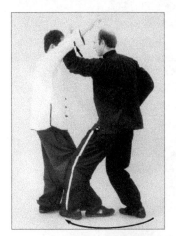 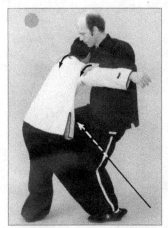 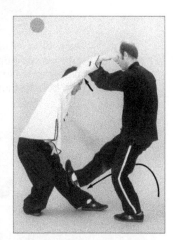

If white does not withdraw his right leg, black's right hand will be able to punch, and his right knee can also kick his stomach. If white steps his right leg back, black can still take advantage and use his right leg to kick white's left knee.

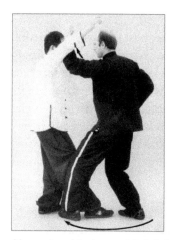 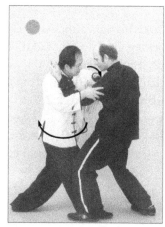

Also, when black uses his left leg to seal white's right leg, his chest is wide open, so white can twist his body and use his left elbow to strike black's chest. This will stop black's right punch and bounce him off balance.

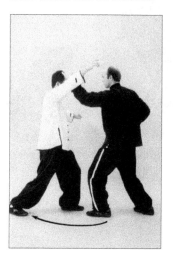 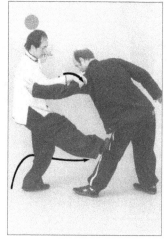

Because the kicking option is mutual, white can use his right leg to kick black's left knee.

4. Deflect and Punch (Ban Chui, 搬捶)

Movements:

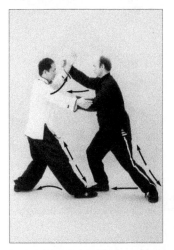 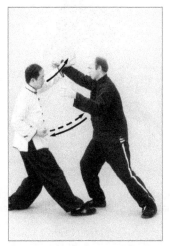 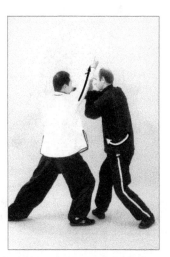

White deflects black's right punch to the side with his left hand, then pulls his right hand back to his waist and punches toward black's chest.

Analysis:

When black punches to his chest, white turns his body to the left and uses his left hand to neutralize the punch and lead it to the side. White also pulls his right hand back to disconnect from black's sticking. White now has a good opportunity to access black's left open door.

Other Options:

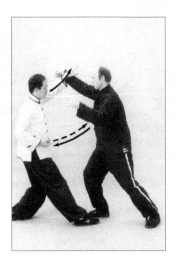 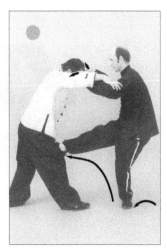

When black finds his punch is blocked, he can hop his rear leg forward, which allows his front leg to be alive for kicking.

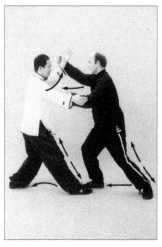 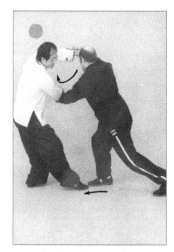 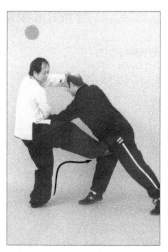

Because white is still sitting back, his right leg is alive and can kick. When he does this, his right hand should coil down to lead black's left hand out of the way, and he should kick with his right leg to the groin or stomach.

5. Step Forward and Left Shoulder Stroke (Shang Bu Zuo Kao, 上步左靠)

Movements:

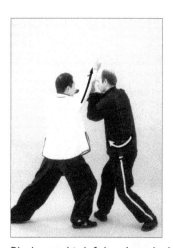 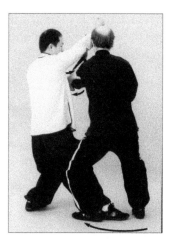

Black uses his left hand to pluck and lead white's elbow up, and at the same time twists his body to his right. He then steps his left leg behind white's right leg to prevent him from withdrawing, and at the same time strikes white's chest with his left elbow.

Analysis:

In order to intercept white's right punch and continue his aggressive attack, black leads white's punch up and to his right. This exposes white's armpit area. He immediately uses his left leg to seal white's withdrawal, and uses his elbow to strike white's chest under the armpit.

Other Options:

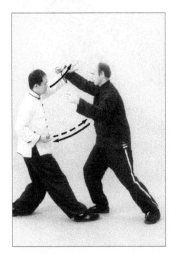 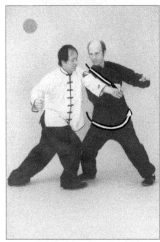 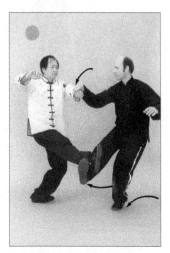

Black can press white's left hand down to stop his right punch, then hop forward and use his right leg to sweep white's right leg.

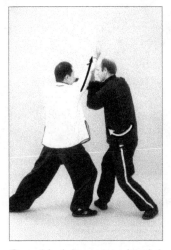 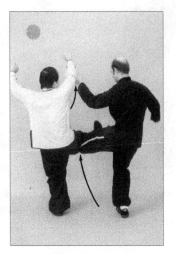

Once black has neutralized the right-hand attack, he can use his left leg to sweep white's right leg and make him fall.

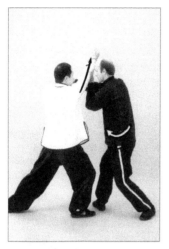 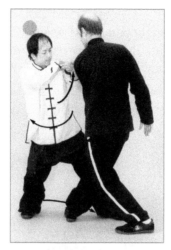 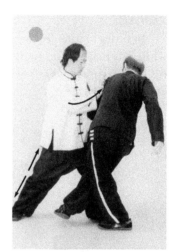

When white finds his right punch neutralized and his armpit area exposed, he can twist his body to the right, scoop up his left arm, and step his left leg behind black's right leg and then press black's left shoulder blade.

6. Strike the Tiger (Right) (You Da Hu, 右打虎)

Movements:

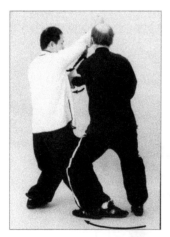 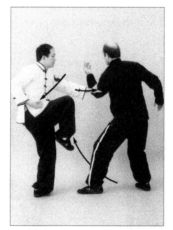 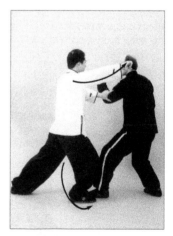

White pushes black's upper arm with his left hand, pulls his right hand back to his waist, and lifts his right leg. He then steps his right leg outside of black's left leg and at the same time uses his right fist to strike black's temple.

Analysis:

In order to stop black's elbow stroke, white first uses his left hand to push black's elbow away, and uses the same motion to withdraw his right leg from black's control. He immediately uses the opportunity to attack.

Other Options:

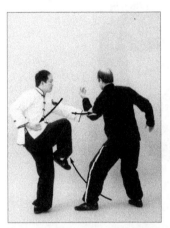 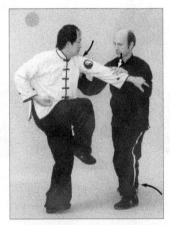 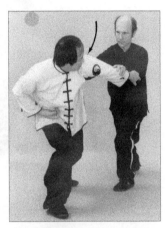

When black's upper arm or elbow is plucked, he is in a bad position. To prevent white's attack and reverse the situation, black can turn his body to the left and immediately follow this with a push to white's left open door.

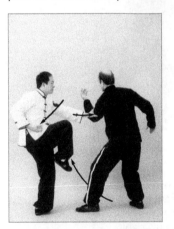 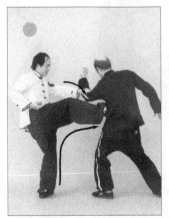 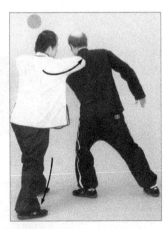

Once white has plucked black's elbow and drawn up his right leg, he is in an advantageous position. He can use his right leg to kick black's left knee or waist. Alternatively, he can use his right elbow to strike black's shoulder blade.

7. Left Elbow Strike (Zuo Zhou Da, 左肘打)

Movements:

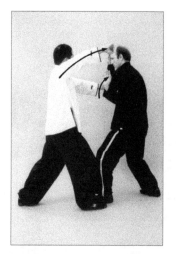 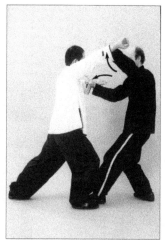

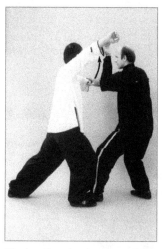 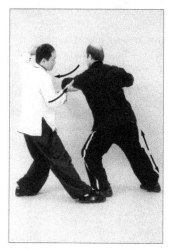

Black twists his body to the right, and at the same time uses his right hand to free his left arm from white's grab. He then twists his body to his left and uses his left hand to intercept white's punch. He immediately twists his body to his right again and uses his elbow to strike white's chest.

Analysis:

When black realizes his left elbow is controlled, he knows he is in danger. He must free his left arm before he can reverse the situation, so he twists his body to his right and pushes white's grip with his right hand. White will naturally use this opportunity to attack because black's whole left side is exposed to attack. Black sees his awkward situation, and immediately uses his left hand to intercept white's strike and reverse the situation, because white's chest is now open to attack. He then uses his left elbow to strike white's chest.

Other Options:

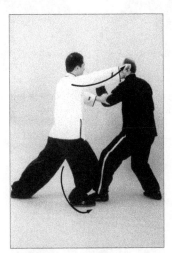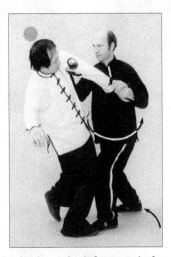

In this situation, black can twist his body to the left instead of to the right, and use both hands to control white's left arm and bounce him off balance.

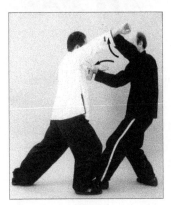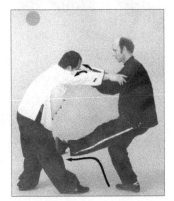

Alternatively, he can use his left leg to kick white's front knee or stomach.

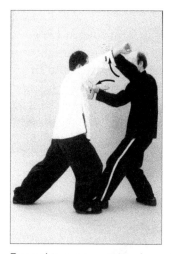 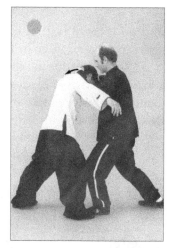 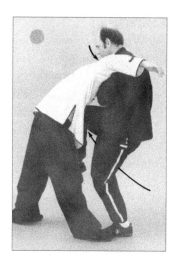

From this same position, he can also use his right hand to hook white's neck and pull him down, and use his right knee to kick white's chest or chin.

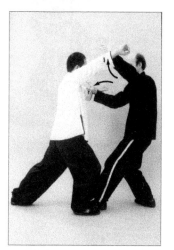 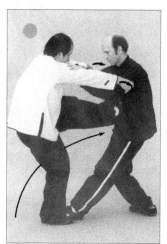

White, from this position, can use his left leg to kick black's stomach.

8. Push to the Left and Right Elbow Stroke (Zuo Tui You Kao, 左推右靠)

Movements:

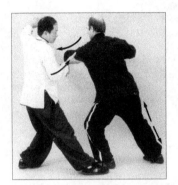 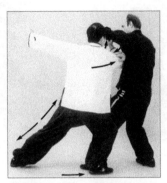

White sits back and uses his right hand to control black's elbow and lead it to his left. He then pushes it up and at the same time uses his right elbow to strike under black's armpit while his right leg hops behind black's left leg to seal his retreat.

Analysis:

When white sees that black is attacking his exposed chest with his elbow, he sits back to yield and at the same time uses his right hand to push the strike to his left. Black will need some time to regain his balance, so white uses this opportunity to continue to push black's elbow up and at the same time strike black with his elbow.

Other Options:

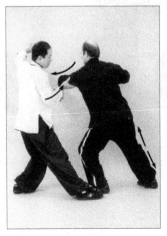 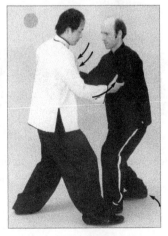

When black's elbow is controlled, he is in danger. He can readjust and step to the right and attack white's left open door. This puts white into a passive, defensive situation.

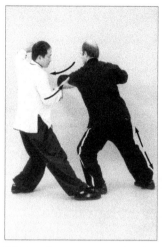 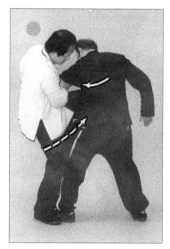 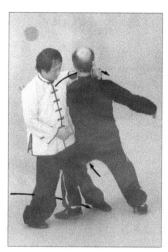

While white controls black's elbow, he is in a temporarily advantageous position. He can use his left knee to kick black's stomach, or else he can step his left leg behind black's left leg, wrap his arm around his neck, and take him down.

9. Withdraw the Step and Strike the Tiger (Left) (Che Bu You Da Hu, 撤步右打虎)

Movements:

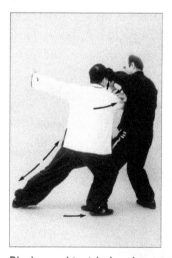 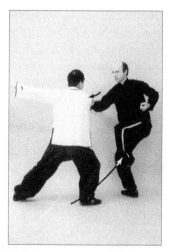 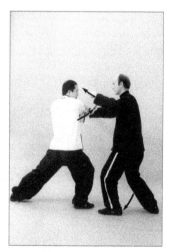

Black uses his right hand to stop white's right elbow stroke, and raises his left leg to evade white's control. He immediately steps his left leg to the outside of white's right leg and strikes toward white's temple with his left fist.

Analysis:

This is the reverse of technique 6. See technique 6, strike the tiger (right) (you da hu, 右打虎), for analysis.

Other Options:

See technique 6, strike the tiger (right) (you da hu, 右打虎).

10. Right Downward Strike (You Xia Chui, 右下捶)

Movements:

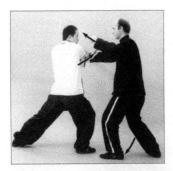
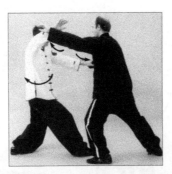
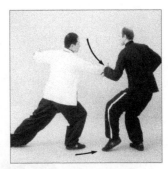

White uses his left hand to push black's right hand away, then sits back and intercepts black's strike with his right hand. He then strikes down with the back of his right fist to black's face.

Analysis:

This is the reverse of technique 7, except that white strikes down instead of using his elbow to strike. See technique 7, left elbow strike (zuo zhou da, 左肘打), for analysis.

Other Options:

See technique 7, left elbow strike (zuo zhou da, 左肘打).

11. Raise Hands to the Up Posture (Ti Shou Shang Shi, 提手上勢)

Movements:

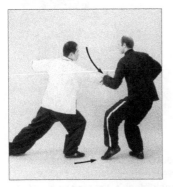
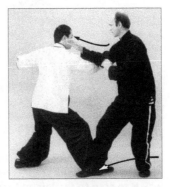

Black sits back into the false stance and uses his left hand to cover white's strike and lead it down. He immediately steps his right leg behind white's right leg and at the same time attacks his neck with a filing strike.

Analysis:

When black sees white strike, he sits back into the false stance and uses his left hand to neutralize the strike downward. He is now in a good position to attack because his left leg can kick and his right hand is ready to strike.

Other Options:

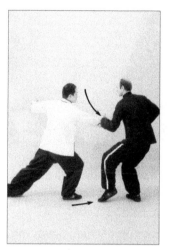 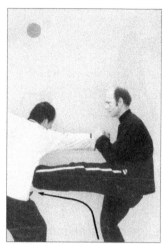

When black neutralizes white's attack and his left leg is empty, black can quickly kick white's waist.

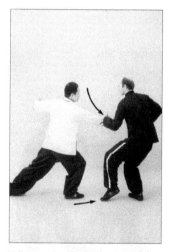 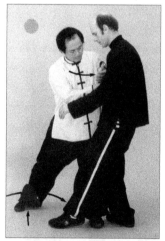

When white's strike has been neutralized, he is in danger, so he must readjust and step to reverse the situation. The best way is to step to the left and attack black's right open door. This renders black's left kick ineffective and puts him in a defensive position.

12. Turn the Body and Push (Zhuan Shen An, 轉身按)

Movements:

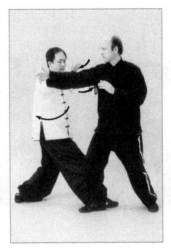

White simply twists his body to his right and uses both hands to control black's right elbow and shoulder, and then pushes forward.

Analysis:

Whenever you are in an awkward situation at short range, the best way out is to twist your body or step to readjust your position. This technique is an example. Simply twisting his body allows white to reverse the situation and lock his opponent's elbow and shoulder.

Other Options:

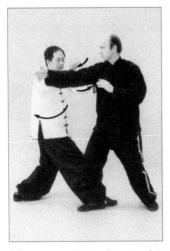 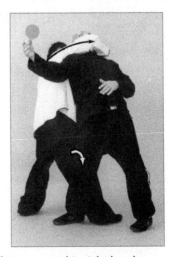

After neutralizing the attack, white can use his right hand to circle around black's neck and pull him down.

13. Right Swinging-Body Strike (You Pie Shen Chui, 右撇身捶)

Movements:

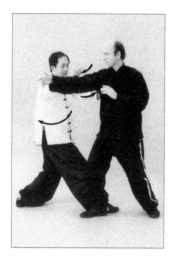 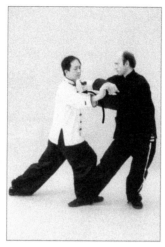 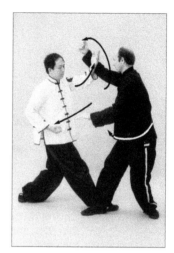

Black uses his left hand to neutralize white's right-hand control, and at the same time twists his body to the right to neutralize white's left-handed push on his shoulder. Black takes this opportunity to strike down to white's face with a backfist.

Analysis:

To escape from this awkward situation, black must neutralize both of white's hands. He therefore neutralizes white's right hand by bending his right arm in and using his left hand to lead white's push away, and at the same time twists his body to the right to neutralize white's left hand. When he twists his body to the right, he also uses this twisting power to strike down toward white's face.

Other Options:

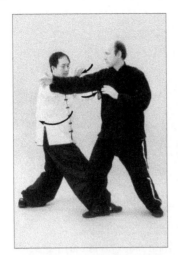
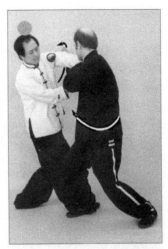
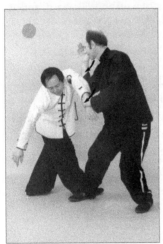
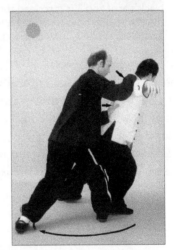

When white has control of black's right elbow and shoulder, black can twist his body to his right and then to the left and use large rollback to execute rollback against white's left arm. He can also step his left leg to the left as he plucks white's right arm, which would put him behind white.

14. Intercept and Punch, One (Ban Chui Yi Shi, 搬捶一勢)

Movements:

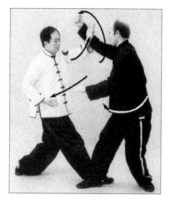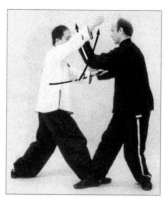

To defend against black's strike, white slides his left arm under black's arm and lifts it to lead the strike up and sideward, and at the same time pulls his right hand back to his waist to prepare to punch. White is now able to punch toward black's chest.

Analysis:

In this short-range situation, coiling and adhering-sticking are very important. If white does not know how to listen and understand black's intention for his right arm, and if he does not know how to stick and coil, he will not be able to neutralize black's strike. Almost at the same time he is neutralizing black's strike, white should punch black's chest with his right hand. Remember: the best time to attack is when your enemy is attacking, because his yi is on attack and not on defense.

Other Options:

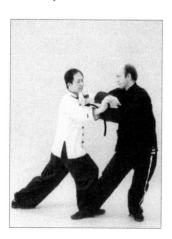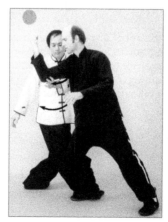

When black twists his body to the right to neutralize white's left-handed push on his shoulder, he has opened white to a backfist attack. White can slide his left hand to black's elbow and push it to his right to stop the attack to his face.

15. Intercept and Punch, Two (Ban Chui Er Shi, 搬捶二勢)

Movements:

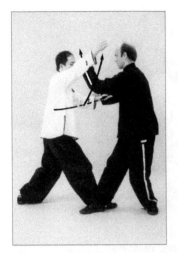 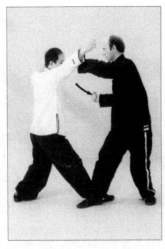 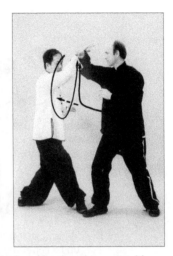

Black intercepts white's punch with his left hand and pulls his right hand back to his waist. He then punches to white's chest. White intercepts black's right punch with a right-hand repel.

Analysis:

After blocking white's punch to his chest, black responds the same way.

Other Options:

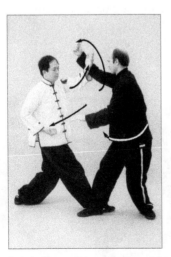 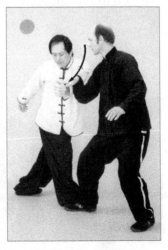

Just before white punches, black can use his right hand to press white's left hand down and to the left, which will put white in an awkward position to punch with his right hand.

16. Wild Horses Shear the Mane (Left) (Zuo Ye Ma Fen Zong, 左野馬分鬃)

Movements:

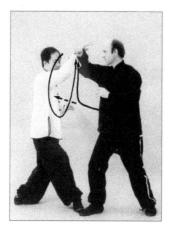 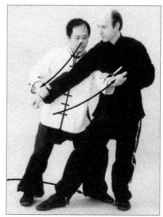

When black punches, white scoops his right hand down and
up to repel the punch, grabs black's right wrist, and twist his
body to the right. He then steps his left leg behind black's right
leg and at the same time places his left upper arm under
black's right armpit, and finally bounces black away.

Analysis:

White changes his strategy and decides to attack through black's right window and
either strikes him under the armpit or else bounces him away. He must be careful to pull
black's wrist downward to prevent black from striking back with his right elbow.

Other Options:

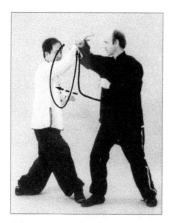 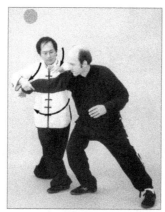 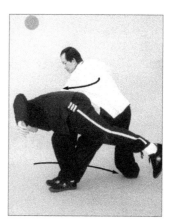

After he has grabbed black's right wrist, white can place his left arm on black's upper arm, and
twist to the right with a circular rend to make black fall.

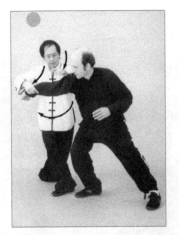 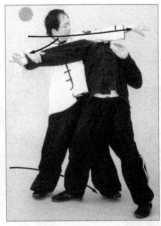

Alternatively, after white has plucked black's right arm
downward, he can wrap black's neck and control black's neck
with his left arm.

17. Strike the Tiger (Right) (You Da Hu, 右打虎)

Movements:

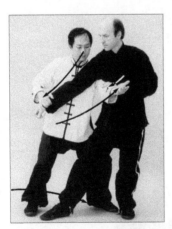 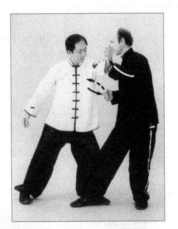

After white steps behind black and places his left upper arm
under black's right armpit, black uses his left hand to push white's
left elbow forward and at the same time pulls his right arm back.
Black then punches white's left armpit with his right fist.

Analysis:

In order to save himself, black must first stop the attack. He therefore pushes white's
left elbow with his left hand and pulls his right hand free. White must release black's
right hand, otherwise both his hands will be crossed in front his chest, and he will be in
danger. When black's hand is free, he punches under white's armpit.

Other Options:

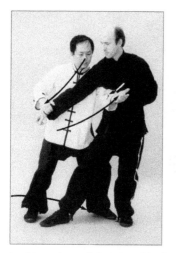 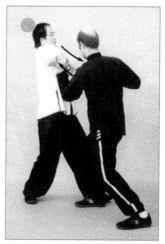 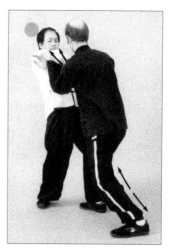

In this awkward situation, black can grab white's right wrist and pull it back while still controlling white's left elbow with his left hand. This sets up an opportunity to cross white's hands in front of his body. However, the most important factor for black in this maneuver is also to step his left leg to the left. From this position, black can use qin na to lock white's arm or just push forward to bounce him away.

18. Turn the Body, Withdraw the Step, and Execute Rollback
(Zhuan Shen Che Bu Lu, 轉身撤步攦)

Movements:

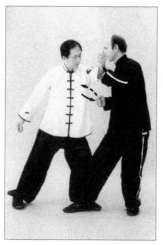 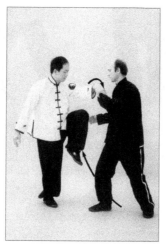 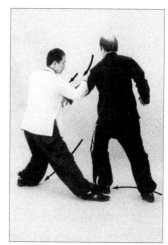

White raises his left knee to seal black's right punch and follows with rollback to black's left arm.

Analysis:

Once black pulls back his right hand, white should sense his danger and react by raising his left knee to seal his side, and at the same time grab black's left hand with his own left hand to set up the next movement. Once black's strike has failed, white steps back and uses this backward momentum to execute rollback against black's left arm.

Other Options:

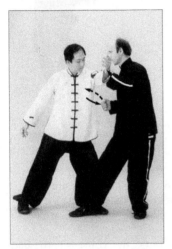 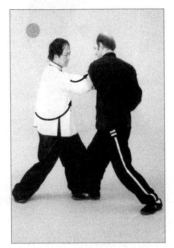 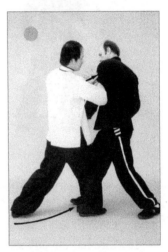

After black uses his left hand to push white's left elbow, white can twist his body to the left and then step his right leg into black's open door and press or shoulder stroke him to make black lose his balance.

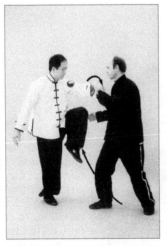 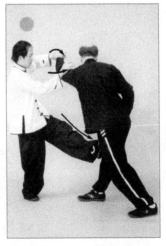

Alternatively, after white raises his left knee to seal black's right punch, he can use his left leg to kick black's right knee or stomach.

19. Step Forward and Press (Left) (Shang Bu Zuo Ji, 上步左擠)

Movements:

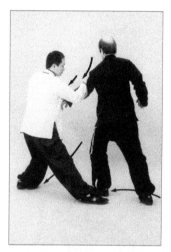 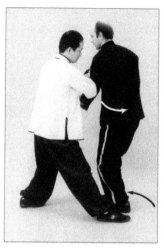 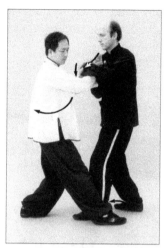

Black steps his right leg forward close to his left leg and at the same time places his right hand on his left arm. He then steps his left leg into white's left open door and presses white's chest.

Analysis:

If white has already sat back to execute rollback, black should not resist but instead should follow the pull so that white feels he is pulling nothing. When white is almost finished pulling, black should redirect the last of white's pulling power to help his press.

Other Options:

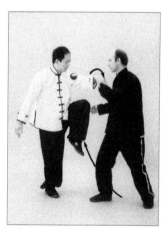 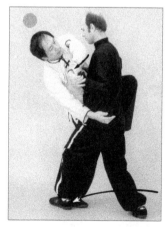

After white raises his left knee to seal black's right punch, if black can catch the right timing just before white steps his left leg backward, black can step his left leg to white's right and push his left hand against white's chest.

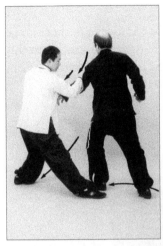 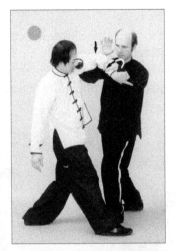 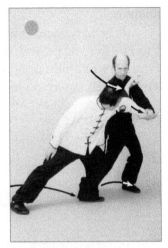

Alternatively, after white pulls down on black's left hand, black can follow the pull and step to readjust his position. He can grab white's left wrist with his left hand and use large rollback on white's left arm.

20. Turn the Body and Press (Left) (Zhuan Shen Zuo Ji, 轉身左擠)

Movements:

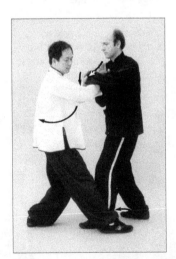 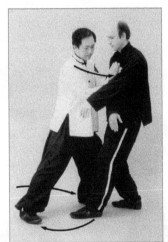

White neutralizes black's press by rotating his body to his right. He quickly readjusts his steps and counters by pressing black's chest from black's right open door.

Analysis:

All the techniques that strike with the elbow, forearm, or shoulder are short-range attacks. How you use your body is crucial in neutralizing such short-range attacks. In this situation, white must turn his body to neutralize the press at the right time, so that he can lead the press into emptiness and also give himself plenty of time to counterattack.

Other Options:

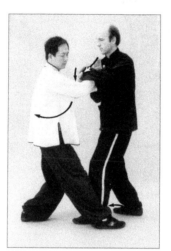 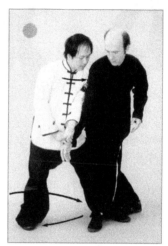

After white neutralizes black's press by rotating his body to his right, white can twist his body to his right, step to readjust his position, and use his shoulder to strike black's shoulder or chest.

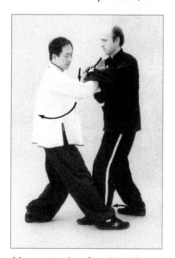 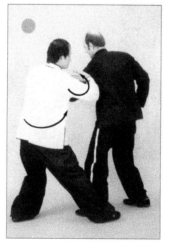 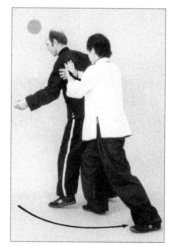

Alternatively, after black's press, white can neutralize the press to his left and then readjust his position to strike black's back.

21. Double Dividing and Heel Kick (Shuang Fen Deng Jiao, 雙分蹬腳)

Movements:

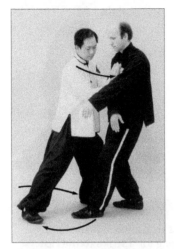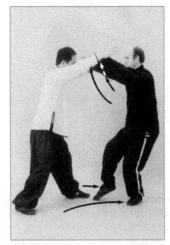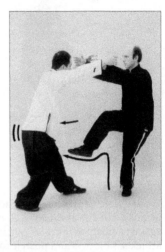

Black steps his left leg back into a false stance to yield to white's press, and at the same time spreads both hands upward to open white's chest. His right leg then kicks white's groin or stomach.

Analysis:

By stepping back, black changes his fighting strategy from short-range fighting into middle range, and also sets up for a kicking attack. As a matter of fact, unless time and space are very short, you can usually evade a press or push by simply stepping back. Therefore, in order to effectively push or press, you must usually first seal and lock the opponent's leg. When you use push or press, your opponent must feel that time is very urgent and he does not have enough time to yield.

Other Options:

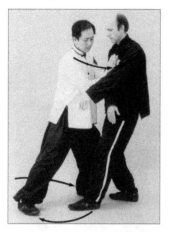 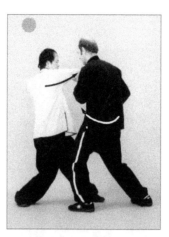 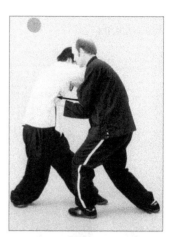

When white presses black, black can neutralize white's press again and return back with a press or push. He can also use large rollback on either of white's arms. These are general reactions against a push or press. A quick and effective solution to a press is to control either of the attacker's elbows and push it to the side. This will create an opening for a strike to the ribs or down to the stomach area.

22. Punch the Groin (Zhi Dang Chui, 指襠捶)

Movements:

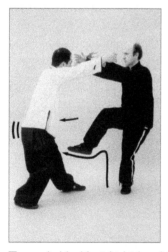 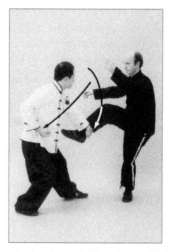 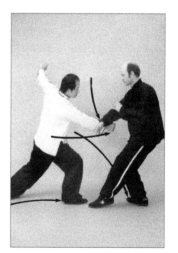

To evade black's right kick, white sits back to yield and uses his left hand to scoop and push the kick aside. He immediately steps his right leg forward to shorten the fighting range and uses his right fist to strike the groin.

Analysis:

White has several options to escape from black's kick. He can intercept the kick as in this technique. He can also pull both hands down to destroy black's balance and force him to stop his kick and regain his balance. White can also attack from the side door to avoid the kick and create the chance for a further attack.

Other Options:

There are many options for white to react to this kick. Here, we will introduce only two examples.

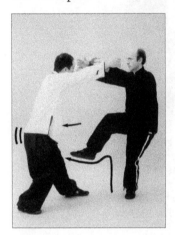 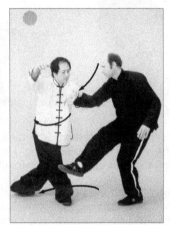 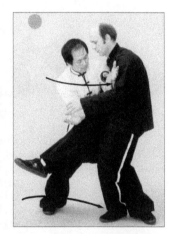

Because both of white's hands are sticking to black's, he can pull black's right hand down to destroy black's balance. In order to save his balance and stability, black must stop his kicking attack and regain his balance. White should use this opportunity, before black regains his stability, to push him or use other techniques to bounce him away.

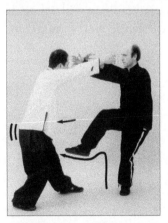 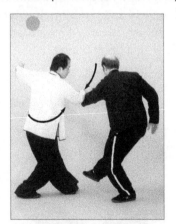 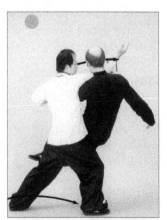

Alternatively, white can evade black's kick by leading down black's left hand and access black's open door or window for an immediate attack. For example, white can press black's right hand down and turn his body to his left, and then step his right leg behind black's left leg and use diagonal flying to bounce black away.

23. Step Forward to Pluck and Rend (Shang Bu Cai Lie, 上步採挒)

Movements:

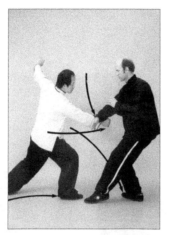 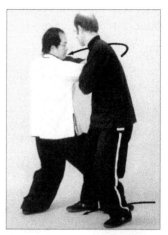

When black finds that his kick is blocked and his groin is going to be attacked, he immediately steps his right leg back and uses his right hand to block down to intercept the groin punch. He then uses his left hand to pluck white's right elbow downward as he steps a short step forward with his left leg, and then steps behind white's right leg with his right leg and simultaneously hooks white's neck with his right arm.

Analysis:

Black must pull his right leg back immediately to avoid having it grabbed. He should also notice that once his kick is in vain, his groin and stomach areas are exposed to attack. Therefore, he steps backward to yield and put himself in a neutral position with white. If he can control white's right arm, he can step forward and either use rend to take him down or else attack his temple with a hook punch.

Other Options:

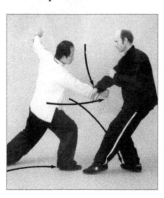 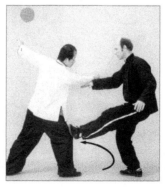

After he has neutralized the groin punch, black can kick white's knee.

24. Fair Lady Weaves with Shuttle, One (Yu Nu Chuan Suo Yi Shi, 玉女穿梭一勢)

Movements:

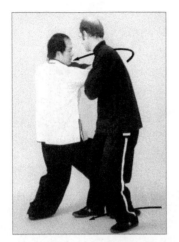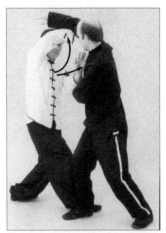

White turns his body to his left and at the same time raises his right arm to lead black's attack upward. White then turns back and leads the motion to his right to expose black's armpit, and at the same time strikes black's armpit.

Analysis:

When black changes from middle range to short range and blocks white from withdrawing with his right leg, white knows he is in an urgent situation. He leads the attack upward, then turns his body to his right to reverse the situation and create an opportunity to attack black's armpit.

Other Options:

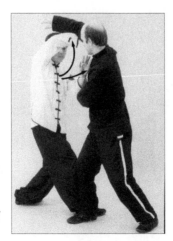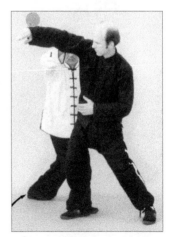

When white raises his arm to stop black's strike, he could step his left leg forward to reach black's right open door and immediately push black off balance.

25. Fair Lady Weaves with Shuttle, Two (Yu Nu Chuan Suo Er Shi, 玉女穿梭二勢)

Movements:

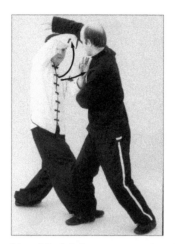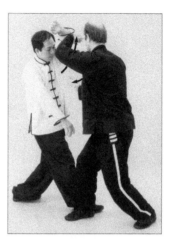

Now black is in an urgent situation. To save himself from white's armpit strike, he turns his body to the right and then the left, and raises his left arm and deflects white's attack. He then strikes white's chest with his right hand.

Analysis:

Because this technique is short range, you usually do not have enough time to readjust your steps to reverse the situation. Therefore, in order to evade the strike, you must use your hand to intercept the attack and at the same time twist your body to neutralize the attack.

Other Options:

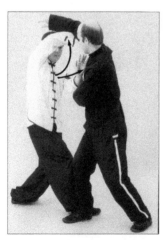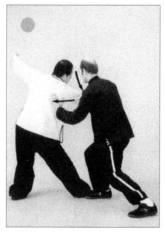

If time allows, black should step his left leg to his left and at the same time pull his right hand down. This will reverse the situation and put him in an advantageous position for a further attack.

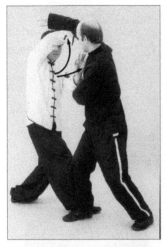
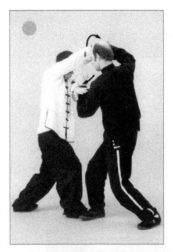
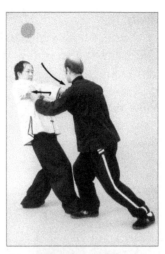

Black can also use his left hand to lead white's left hand upward and at the same time use his right hand to grab white's right wrist. He can then cross white's arms in front of his body and push white off balance.

26. White Crane Spreads Its Wings (Bai He Liang Chi, 白鶴亮翅)

Movements:

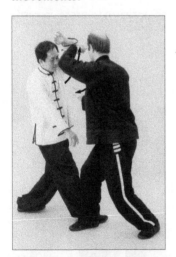
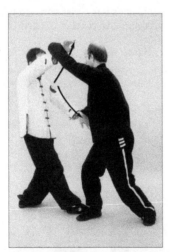
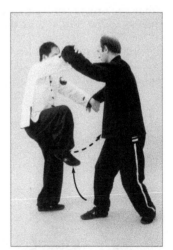

White sits back into a false stance and at the same time leads black's left hand up with his right hand, and neutralizes black's right hand downward with his left hand. He then kicks with his right leg to black's groin or stomach.

Analysis:

Because both white and black are sticking with each other, it is difficult for either side to attack successfully. Therefore, white changes his strategy by spreading black's hands and kicking.

Other Options:

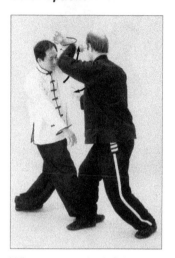 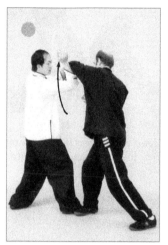 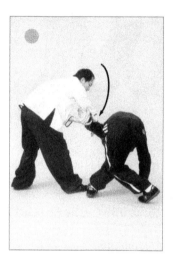

White can use his left hand to grasp black's left wrist and use his right forearm to press upward, and then circle down to use qin na control on black's left arm.

27. Left Shoulder Stroke (Zuo Kao, 左靠)

Movements:

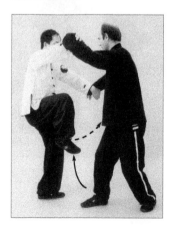 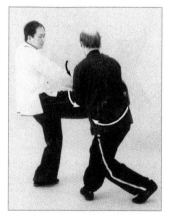 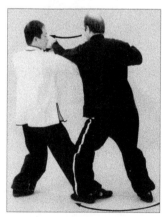

In order to evade white's kick, black turns his body to his right and at the same time uses his right hand to lead the kick to his right and his left hand to press white's right arm down. Black then steps forward and does a left diagonal flying or shoulder stroke.

Analysis:

Black is in a very exposed position, so in addition to pulling his left arm down and to his right to stop the kick, he also turns his body out of the way and coils his right arm over white's arm and down to help deflect the kick.

Other Options:

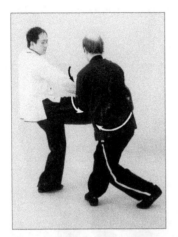 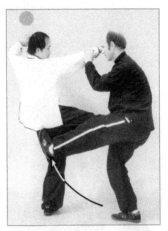

Once black has neutralized the kick, and before white's right leg returns to the floor, black can use a left low lift-hook kick (di qiao) to kick white's tailbone.

28. Execute Rollback against the Shoulder (Lu Bi, 擺臂)

Movements:

In order to regain stability after his kick, white pulls his right leg back and steps down, and uses his left hand to stop black's left-arm attack. White circles his right arm to the outside of black's left upper arm as he moves his right leg from the inside of black's left leg to the outside, and then uses rollback on black's left arm.

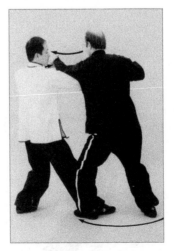 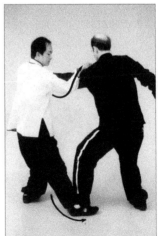

Analysis:

Once white's kick is neutralized, he is in a bad position. To avoid having his kicking leg hooked or grabbed, he has to pull it back as soon as possible, and then he has to worry about his upper body being exposed to attack. Unless he immediately stabilizes his position with both feet on the ground, he will probably be quickly bounced away. Unless time is very short, the best reaction to black's attack is for white to turn his body to his right and step his left leg to his left. This will give him a better position for his attack.

Other Options:

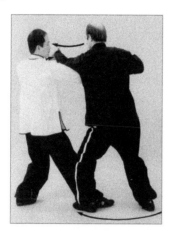 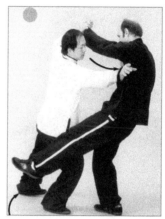

After white uses rollback on black's left arm, white can step his left leg to black's right open door and press black's left arm forward, and at the same time use his right arm to execute wardoff against black.

29. Turn the Body to Rend the Shoulder (Zhuan Shen Lie Bi, 轉身捯臂)

Movements:

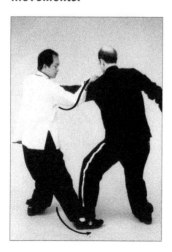 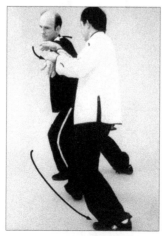

Once white has caught black's arm, he steps his left leg to his rear to execute a circular rend on black.

Analysis:

To prevent black from countering with a press, and also to keep his advantageous position, white uses circular rend to swing black around to destroy his balance or cause him to resist in a way that could be utilized.

Other Options:

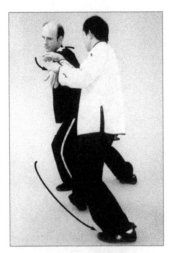
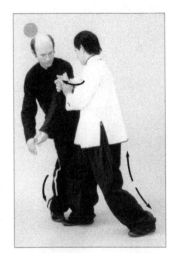

White can start pulling black in a circular rend, and when black senses white's intention and steps to follow the pull, white can immediately borrow his momentum and bounce him backward. This is the trick of borrowing jing.

30. Turn the Body to Execute Rollback (Zhuan Shen Lu, 轉身攦)

Movements:

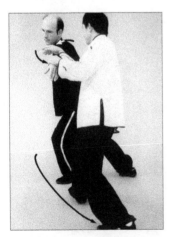
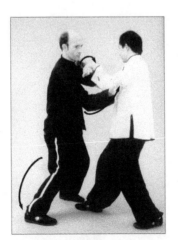
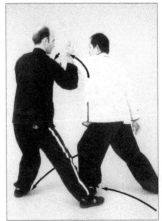

Black does not resist white's pull. Instead, he reverses the situation by following white's pulling power. He steps his right leg forward and at the same time turns his left hand to grab white's left arm, and controls white's elbow with his right arm. He then steps his left leg back and uses rollback on white's left arm.

Analysis:

The natural reaction to a circular rend is to resist, but your opponent can change his attack and push you as you pull, knocking you off balance so that you are open to attack. It is far better to follow his attack by stepping forward, because this will let you readjust the situation and find an opening for an attack.

Other Options:

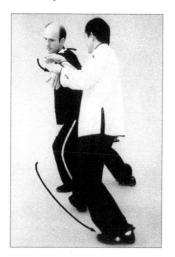 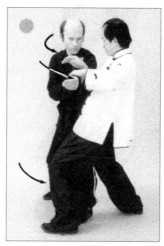

When black's opponent is pulling him, he can readjust the pulling direction slightly toward his opponent and strike him with either shoulder stroke or press.

31. Two Winds Pass Through the Ears (Shuang Feng Guan Er, 雙風貫耳)

Movements:

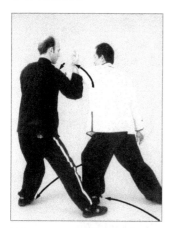 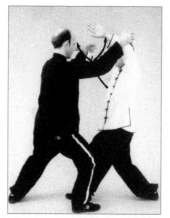 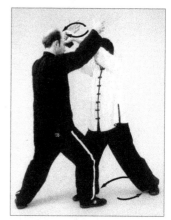

White steps his left leg forward to follow black's rollback power. He uses his right hand to remove black's left hand and his left hand to repel black's right hand. White then adjusts his legs and at the same time attacks black's temples with both fists.

Analysis:

White does not resist but instead follows the rollback power and steps into a firm stance. In this example, he uses both hands to spread out and nullify black's arms, and immediately attacks.

Other Options:

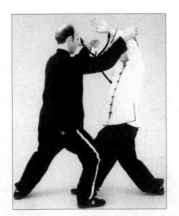 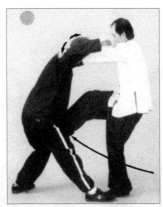

Two winds pass through the ears is a common counter against a rollback press or shoulder stroke. Spreading the opponent's arms gives you the option of kicking to the groin or stomach.

32. Double Push (Shuang An, 雙按)

Movements:

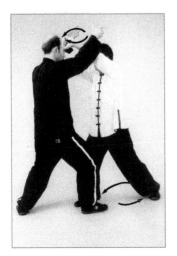 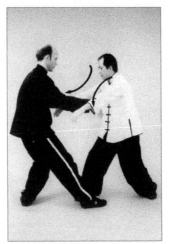 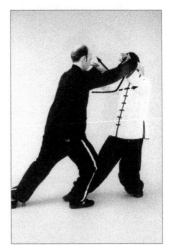

In order to save himself from white's attack, black sits back to yield and at the same time presses both hands downward and spreads them to the sides. He then immediately uses both hands to push white's chest.

Analysis:

This technique is a typical example of the application of adhering-sticking. A natural reaction when you are sticking is to redirect the opponent's attack to a position that is disadvantageous to him. There is another easy and effective solution against a double-hand strike, and that is to neutralize the attack to the side. This allows you to open the side window for an attack or even enter from the open door directly.

Other Options:

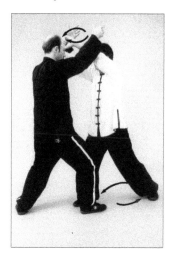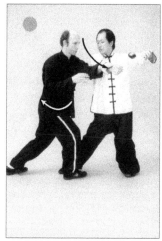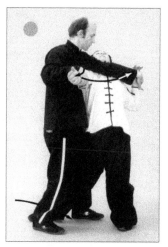

Black can press his left hand down to open white's upper window, and step his left leg behind white's right leg as he attacks white's neck with his left arm.

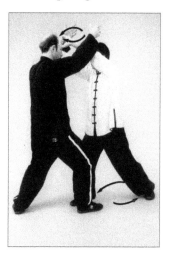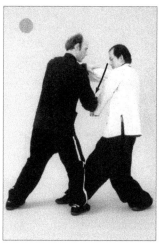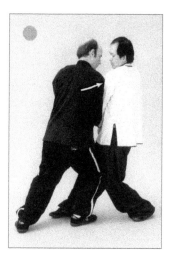

Black could also use his right hand to neutralize the attack to his left and then follow with a shoulder stroke.

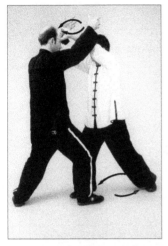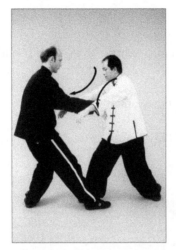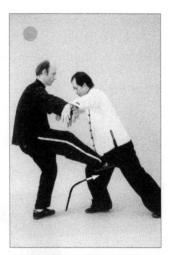

Alternatively, if black neutralizes the attack downward with both hands, he can easily and quickly use his right leg to kick white's groin.

33. Single Whip (Dan Bian, 單鞭)

Movements:

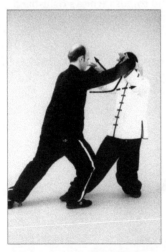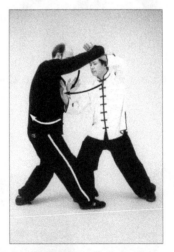

When black pushes toward white's chest, white sits back and at the same time neutralizes the attack up and to the sides. He immediately pushes black's chest with his right hand while still sticking to black's right hand with his left hand.

Analysis:

Like the last technique, this is also an example of neutralization coming from adhering-sticking. Naturally, white can also neutralize to the side and follow with a strike.

Other Options:

See technique 32, double push (shuang an, 雙按).

34. Right Push (You Tui, 右推)

Movements:

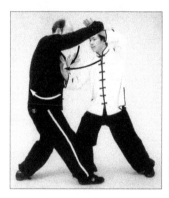

Black turns his body to his right and at the same time uses his left hand to push white's right-hand attack to the right.

Analysis:

Because white's strike is short and sudden, the quickest and most effective way for black to defend is to turn his body and use adhere-stick neutralization with his left hand.

Other Options:

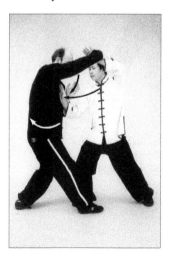
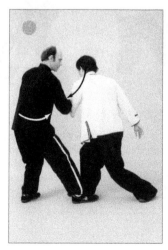

After black pushes white's attack to his right, he can then press down with his right hand and turn his body to his left. This will neutralize the attack and also give him an opportunity to access white's left open door.

35. File the Shoulder (Right) (You Cuo Bi, 右挫臂)

Movements:

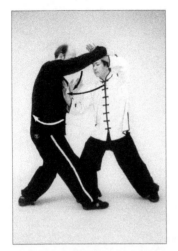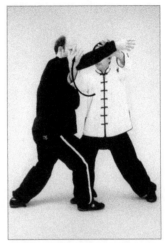

When white finds his right-hand attack is neutralized, he changes his strategy and continues his attack by locking black's right arm in order to break it.

Analysis:

This technique is applicable only if black's right hand is still sticking with white's left hand. When black neutralizes the attack to his right, if he also pulls his right hand back, he will not give white the opportunity to lock his arm.

Other Options:

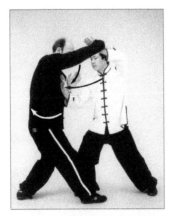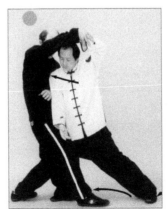

Instead of locking black's right arm, white can hop forward and use his shoulder to strike black's chest from his left open door.

36. Follow the Posture and Push (Shun Shi An, 順勢按)

Movements:

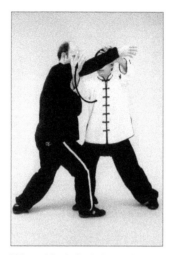 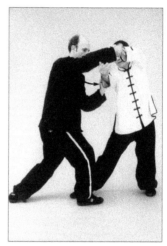

When black finds his right arm is in danger, he uses his left hand to push white's right elbow forward and at the same time pulls his right hand back.

Analysis:

Whenever your arm is about to be locked, the first reaction should be to bend your arm so that it will be difficult to lock or break. This is the most natural reaction for most people. In this case black also "follows white's posture" (i.e., as white reaches for his arm, black pushes white's arm past him).

Other Options:

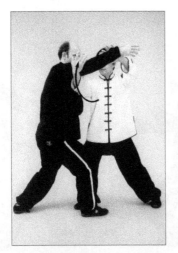
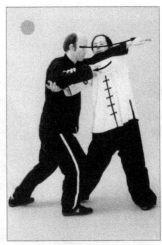
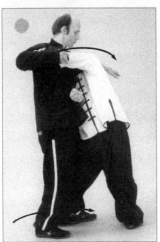
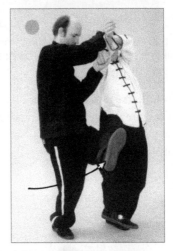

Black can pull back and bend his right arm first to resist the breaking, and at the same time use his left arm to lock white's neck. This puts white in a very bad situation and forces him to do something to save himself. Black can also use his left leg to sweep white's right leg. As white falls, he will naturally release black's arm.

37. Neutralize and Strike with Right Palm (Hua Da You Zhang, 化打右掌)

Movements:

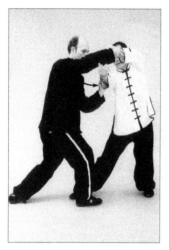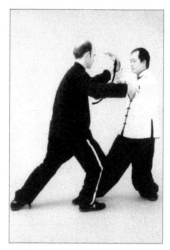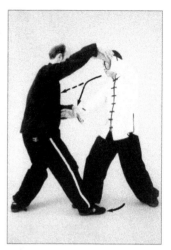

White turns his body to his right and at the same time neutralizes black's push with his right hand. He then uses his right hand to push black's chest again.

Analysis:

Many of the adhere-stick neutralizations used in this fighting set are not necessarily the best techniques for a real fight. However, adhere-stick neutralizing is still the foundation of taijiquan, so they are included for training purposes and also to allow the practice to continue smoothly.

Other Options:

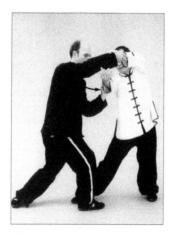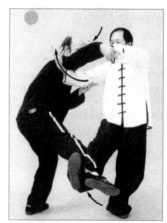

White can follow black's push and sit back, and at the same time use his right leg to sweep black's right leg to destroy his root.

38. Neutralize and Push (Hua Tui, 化推)

Movements:

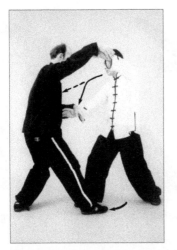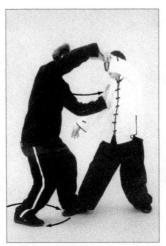

Black again uses his left hand to neutralize white's right-hand attack downward. As he does this, he steps back a half step with his right foot. Black immediately steps forward with his left leg and strikes white's chest with his left hand.

Analysis:

Because the attack starts from very close, black steps his right leg back half a step to help him avoid it. Once he has neutralized the push, he must step his left leg forward, which gives him the most stable position for his strike.

Other Options:

As in previous examples, black can press his right hand down and to his left, or he can sweep his right leg against white's right leg to stop white's punch. He can also use his right leg to kick white's groin.

39. Neutralize and Strike with Right Elbow (Hua Da You Zhou, 化打右肘)

Movements:

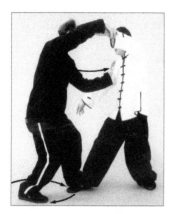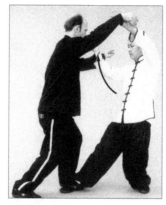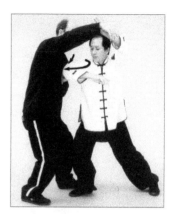

Again, white neutralizes black's push to his right. Because this time black's left leg is forward, white strikes black's chest with his elbow.

Analysis:

In a fight, whenever your opponent's right leg is forward, your right leg is usually also forward. When one has his left leg forward, and the other his right, both persons are more open to attack. Normally, if you are more skillful with your right hand, you would like to have your right leg forward so that your right hand has greater reach and is more alive. Naturally, you will sometimes encounter an opponent who is skillful with his left hand while you prefer using your right hand. In this case, your right foot is forward while his left foot is forward. Under these conditions, your fighting strategy will be different. This will be discussed more fully in the last chapter.

Other Options:

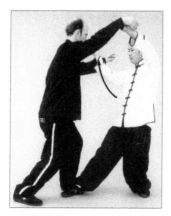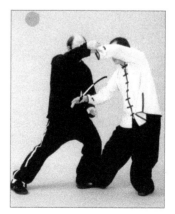

White can cover black's push from the outside instead of neutralizing it from the inside.

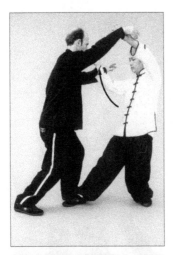 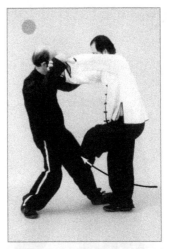

After deflecting black's punch, white could also use his left leg to kick black's front knee.

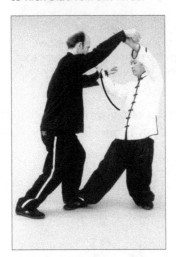 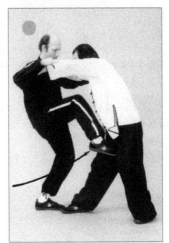

Immediately after his push is deflected, black could use his right leg to kick white's groin.

40. Pluck and Rend (Cai Lie, 採挒)

Movements:

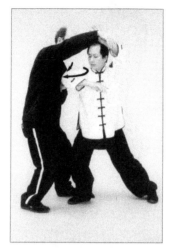 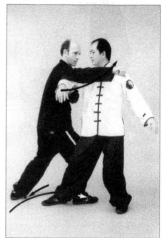

Black uses his left hand to control and push white's elbow strike to the right, and then steps his right leg behind white's right leg while circling white's neck with his right arm.

Analysis:

As mentioned before, the best way to stop an elbow stroke is to control the elbow or upper arm. When white is executing this technique, he should be wary of a possible attack from black's right knee.

Other Options:

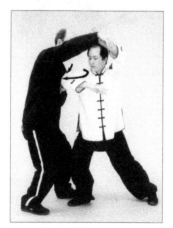 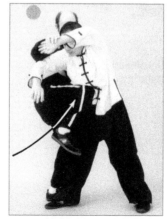

Black can press his left hand to his right and turn his body to the right to avoid being struck, and then follow with a knee kick.

41. Exchange Steps and Execute Rollback (Huan Bu Lu, 換步掘)

Movements:

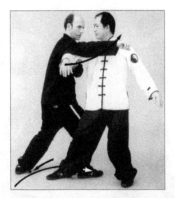 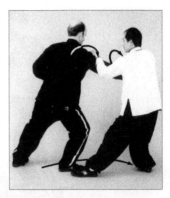

Before black's right arm circles his neck, white withdraws by stepping his right leg backward. As he steps, he plucks black's right wrist back with his right hand and, controlling the elbow with his left hand, executes rollback.

Analysis:

In this technique, white has been placed in a bad position. If black is skillful and knows to use his right leg to seal white's right leg, white will have difficulty escaping from his rend. If you find you are in such an awkward situation, the first reaction should be to use your left hand to stop black's right arm from circling your neck. This will give you more time and allow you to escape from the control of his right leg more easily.

Other Options:

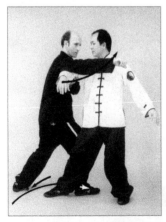 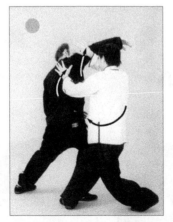 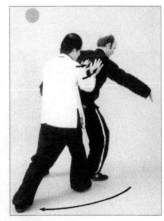

If white finds he cannot withdraw his right leg, he can use his right forearm to lift up against black's armpit to neutralize his arm. He should then step his left leg to his left, which will give him the opportunity to attack black's back from his right open door.

42. Step Forward and Press (Shang Bu Ji, 上步擠)

Movements:

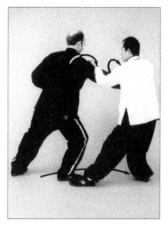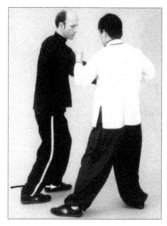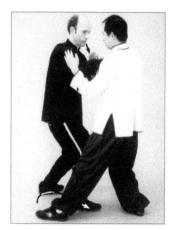

Black steps his left leg forward and then steps his right leg into white's right open door and presses white's chest.

Analysis:

See technique 19, step forward and press (left) (shang bu zuo ji, 上步左擠).

Other Options:

See technique 19, step forward and press (left) (shang bu zuo ji, 上步左擠).

43. Exchange Steps and Execute Rollback (Huan Bu Lu, 換步搌)

Movements:

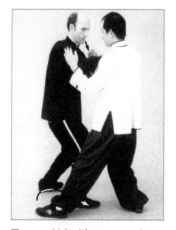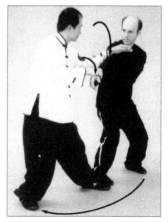

To avoid black's press, white steps his right leg to his rear and uses rollback again.

Analysis:

In practice, press and rollback can be used against each other. The key to success is to attack in the right direction. This training is discussed in the last chapter.

Other Options:

See chapter 3-5 on pushing-hands training for rollback.

44. Strike the Tiger (Right) (You Da Hu, 右打虎)

Movements:

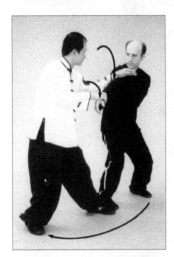 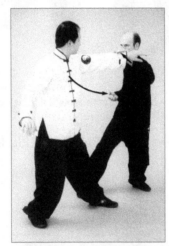 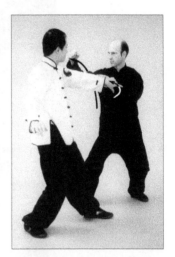

This time, black will not press again because he knows that white expects him to. Instead, he frees his right arm by pulling it back as he pushes white's arm with his left arm. He then strikes white's temple with a right circular strike.

Analysis:

After black frees his right arm, if the distance is short he should use strike the tiger to attack the head. If the distance is too great for this, he should attack under the armpit. White should therefore be careful to protect his face and armpit area. However, white's most vulnerable area is his left knee, which black can kick with his right leg.

Other Options:

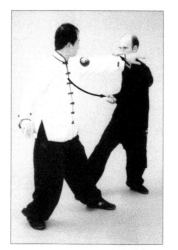 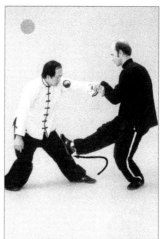

After he pushes white's left arm forward, black can use his right leg to kick white's left knee.

45. Turn the Body, Step Backward, and Execute Rollback (Zhuan Shen Che Bu Lu, 轉身撤步攦)

Movements:

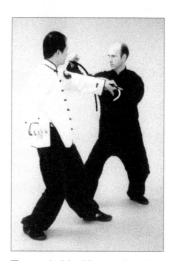 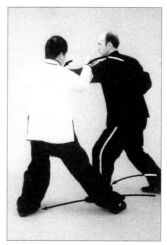

To evade black's punch, white uses his left hand to pluck black's left wrist and turn his body. He then steps his left leg back and uses his right hand on black's elbow to rollback black's left arm.

Analysis:

A principle of taijiquan fighting is that whenever your enemy punches you with one hand, if you can pull his other hand, you will automatically neutralize his attack. This technique is a typical example.

Other Options:

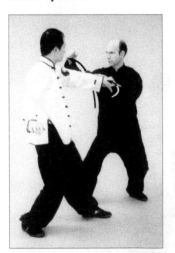 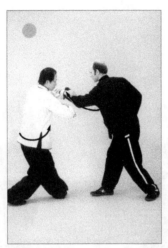 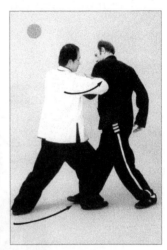

White can also neutralize black's attack by pushing black's left hand to black's right, and then stepping his right leg into black's left open door and striking him with his right shoulder or forearm. Alternatively, he can use his right leg to kick black's groin.

46. Step Forward and Press to the Left (Shang Bu Zuo Ji, 上步左擠)

Movements:

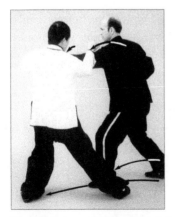 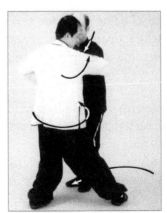

Black follows white's rollback by stepping his left leg forward. He immediately moves his right leg to his left leg and presses white's chest.

Analysis:

See technique 19, step forward and press (left) (shang bu zuo ji, 上步左擠).

Other Options:

See technique 19, step forward and press (left) (shang bu zuo ji, 上步左擠).

47. Return with Press (Hui Ji, 回擠)

Movements:

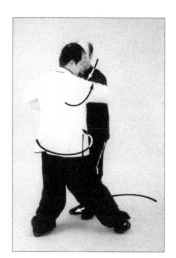 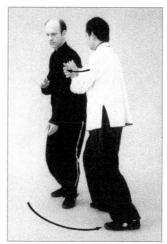

White turns his body to his left to neutralize the press and at the same time moves his left leg to his rear. He then presses black's shoulder blade from his left open door.

Analysis:

The key to avoid being pressed is to readjust your steps before your opponent's press jing is out. Therefore, once you sense the awkward situation, you should already be prepared for what is going to happen and be ready to act.

Other Options:

White can turn his body to his right to neutralize the press and follow with a press as in technique 20, turn the body and press (left) (zhuan shen zuo ji, 轉身左擠).

48. Exchange Steps and Shoulder Stroke (Right) (Huan Bu You Kao, 换步右靠)

Movements:

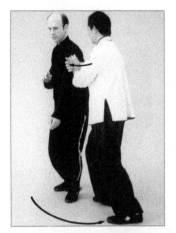 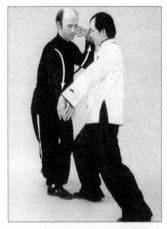 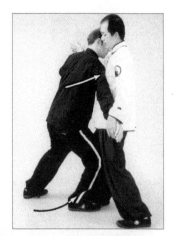

To avoid being pressed, black quickly turns his body to his left as he spreads his arms, lifting white's right arm with his left hand and leading white's left arm down with his right hand. He then steps his right leg into white's left open door and strikes white's exposed chest with his shoulder.

Analysis:

To counter a shoulder blade press, turn your body just before the opponent's press jing is out. This neutralizes the press by leading it into emptiness. Most of the time, the short-range jing can only be neutralized by turning or twisting the body. You usually don't have the time or space to use your hand or arm. Therefore, you should investigate the right timing and techniques for using your body to neutralize short-range attacks.

Other Options:

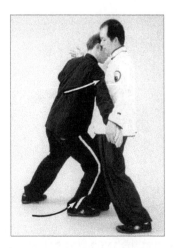 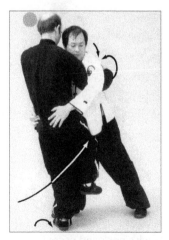

Right after black's shoulder stroke, he can use both hands to hold white's body and hop forward and kick white's groin with his right knee.

49. Turn the Body to Fly Diagonally (Zhuan Shen Xie Fei Shi, 轉身斜飛勢)

Movements:

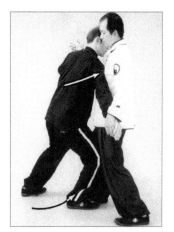
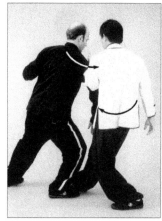
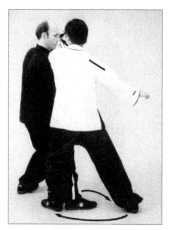

White neutralizes the strike with his left arm as he sits back and turns his body to the right. He then switches legs so that his left leg seals black's right leg, and at the same time strikes black's neck with his left arm.

Analysis:

White must be careful when he uses this attack because his groin is open to attack from black's right hand. To avoid this, he should seal black's right elbow with his right hand. In short-range fighting like this, both sides should be wary of knee attacks. Also, each side can sweep the other's leg to destroy his root.

Other Options:

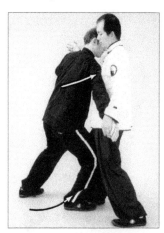
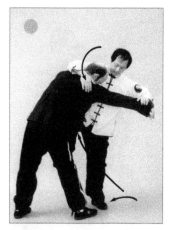
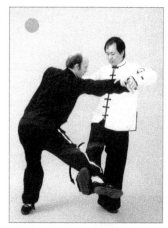

When black uses his shoulder to strike white's chest, white can use his right hand to circle black's neck and press it down, and at the same time hop kick black's groin or stomach. Alternatively, he can sweep his right leg against black's right leg to upset black's root and stop the shoulder stroke before it starts.

50. Right Elbow Strike (You Zhou Da, 右肘打)

Movements:

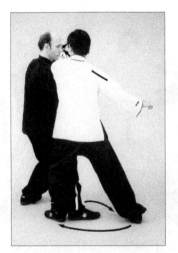 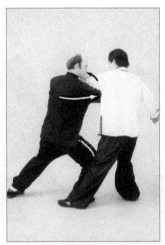

Black sits back and pushes white's elbow with his left hand to stop his attack, and then strikes him under his armpit with his right elbow.

Analysis:

Because the range is so short, black must be careful to stop the attack early. He must also shift his weight back to avoid being bounced.

Other Options:

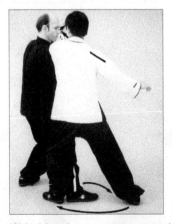 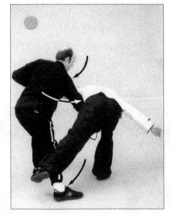

If black's right arm is not properly sealed, he can swing his hand down to strike white's groin. Because his right leg is inside of white's left leg and solid, he can also sweep his right leg backward as he presses his right shoulder down to destroy white's root.

51. Turn the Body for Rooster Standing on One Leg
(Zhuan Shen Jin Ji Du Li, 轉身金雞獨立)

Movements:

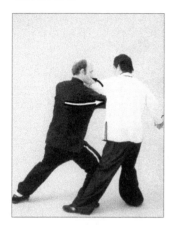
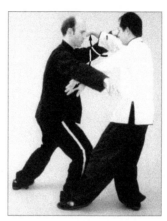
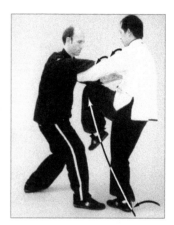

White uses his right hand to free his left hand and at the same time uses his left hand to guide black's right arm to the side. He then hops forward and kicks black's stomach with his left knee.

Analysis:

As mentioned before, whenever you spread the opponent's arms, you are in a good position to kick. This technique is a typical example. If black has grabbed white's left wrist tightly, white will have difficulty freeing his arm. In such a situation, the quickest way for white to defend himself from black's elbow would be for him to stop the elbow with his right hand. Alternatively, he can turn his body to the left and at the same time pull black's left wrist. This will stop the attack and put the opponent in a defensive position.

Other Options:

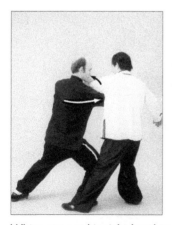
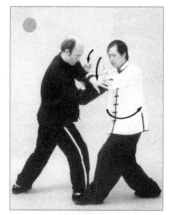
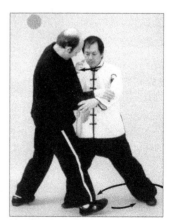

White can use his right hand to push black's attacking elbow at the same time he turns his body and pulls black's left hand to his left. White can then execute wardoff with his right arm, causing black to lose his balance.

52. Downward Neutralization (Xia Hua, 下化)

Movements:

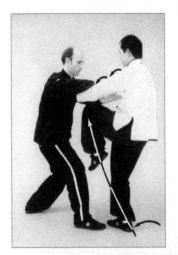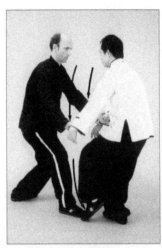

When black finds that he is in danger from white's kick, he uses both hands to pull white's arms down.

Analysis:

The best way to stop a kick is to pull the opponent's arm down. This will destroy his balance and stop the kick.

Other Options:

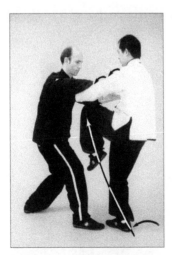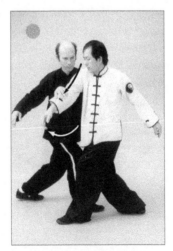

Instead of pulling down, black can pull one of white's arms to the side to stop the kick.

53. Heel Kick (Deng Jiao, 蹬腳)

Movements:

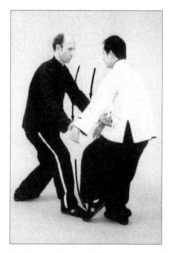 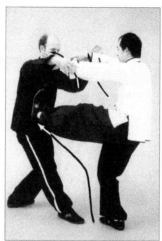

White suddenly lifts both hands and attacks black's stomach with a left heel kick.

Analysis:

When black presses white's arms down, he has neutralized white's attack. Black's yi will now be on attacking. White uses this opportunity to surprise kick black. Usually, if black is a beginner, white's strategy will be successful.

Other Options:

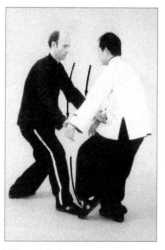 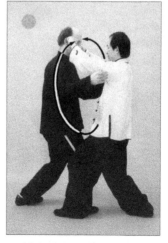

When black presses white's arms, white can use this pressing power and circle up to strike black's temples.

54. Turn the Body, Step Forward, and Strike
(Zhuan Shen Shang Bu Kao, 轉身上步靠)

Movements:

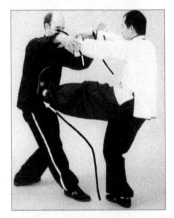 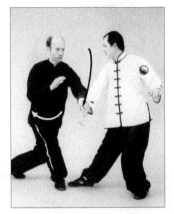 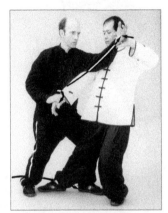

To neutralize white's kick, black twists his body to his right to avoid the kick, and also uses his left hand to push white's hand to the right in order to turn him and deflect the kick. He continues to push his left hand down and steps his left leg behind white's right leg. While doing this, his right hand grabs white's wrist and his left elbow strikes white's chest.

Analysis:

This is a good move for black. It not only neutralizes the threatening kick, but it also puts white in a defensive position.

Other Options:

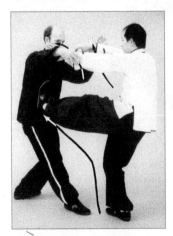 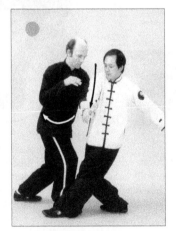 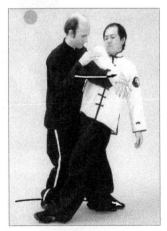

To avoid white's kick, black can twist his body to his right and press his left hand down and then step in and press white's chest while white's left leg is rerooting. This move will bounce white off balance.

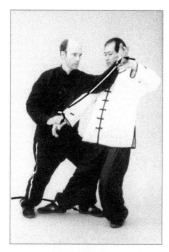 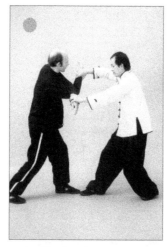 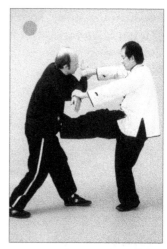

White can push his left hand forward while he is twisting his body to his right and use his right hand to grab black's right wrist. He can then cross black's arms in front of his body and then hop forward and use his right leg to kick black's stomach.

55. Execute Rollback against Left Arm (Lu Zuo Bi, 掤左臂)

Movements:

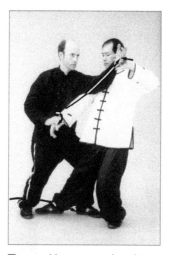 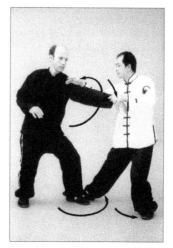

To avoid being struck, white stops black's elbow strike with his left hand as he pulls his right arm free. He then places his right hand above black's elbow and steps his right leg behind black's left leg. He finally steps his left leg back and does rollback on black's arm.

Analysis:

See technique 28, execute rollback against the shoulder (lu bi, 擺臂).

Other Options:

See technique 28, execute rollback against the shoulder (lu bi, 擺臂).

56. Turn the Body and Right Kick (Zhuan Shen You Fen Jiao, 轉身右分腳)

Movements:

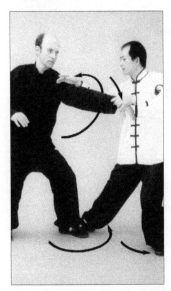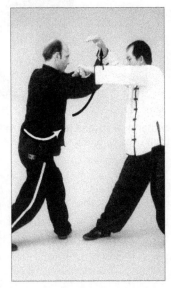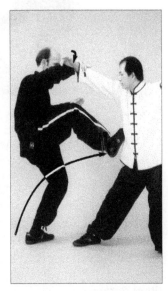

Black turns his body to his left and at the same time pushes white's right hand up with his right hand. Black then kicks white's waist with his right leg.

Analysis:

In a real fight, black's best targets would be white's knee or groin because they would be harder to protect. Of course, white's best reaction to a kick would be to pull down black's hand.

Other Options:

Black can use the usual options against large rollback.

57. Double Dividing and Embrace the Knee (Right)
(Shuang Fen You Lou Xi, 雙分右摟膝)

Movements:

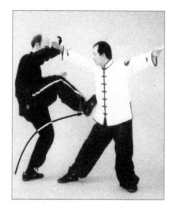 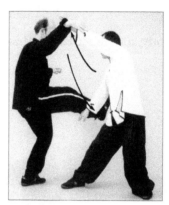

White uses his left hand to spread to the left and free his right hand, which he then uses to block black's kick.

Analysis:

To use your hand or arm to intercept a kick is not the best policy. Kicks can be very powerful and can injure your arm. Unless absolutely necessary, you should not use your hand to block a powerful kick. In a situation like this, if white's right hand can hook black's wrist, he can pull it down to solve the problem. If black is not controlling white's hand, white will not be able to pull it down, so he should step back to evade the kick.

Other Options:

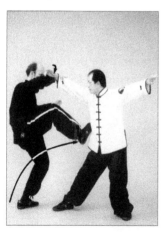 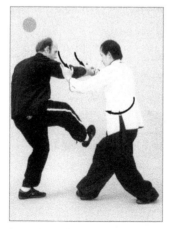 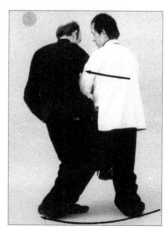

White can turn his body to his right and use his right hand to grab black's right hand and pull it down. He can then step his left leg forward behind black's left leg to seal black's retreat and bounce black away. Alternatively, he can kick black's tailbone with his left leg.

58. Turn the Body and Left Kick (Zhuan Shen Zuo Fen Jiao, 轉身左分腳)

Movements:

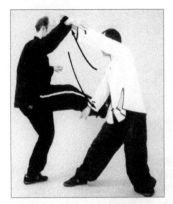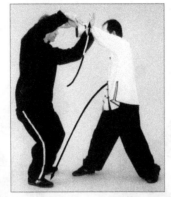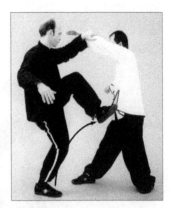

Black puts his right leg down and twists his body to his right while using his left hand to push away white's left hand. He then kicks white's left waist with his left leg.

Analysis:

Whenever your leg is blocked, you should withdraw and restabilize yourself immediately, otherwise your opponent can take the opportunity to kick your tailbone or strike you to bounce you away.

Other Options:

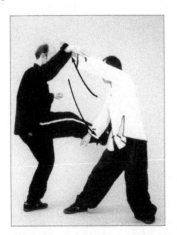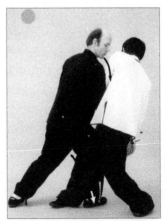

Once black finds his kick blocked, he can step his right leg forward and behind white's right leg and at the same time use his right hand to push white's left hand down. This will put white in an awkward position.

59. Double Dividing and Embrace the Knee (Left)
(Shuang Fen Zuo Lou Xi, 雙分左摟膝)

Movements:

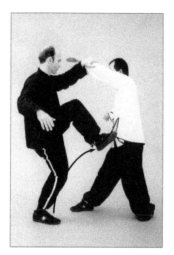 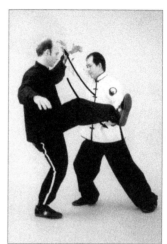

White uses his right hand to push away black's left hand and at the same time uses his left hand to block black's left kick.

Analysis:

See technique 57, double dividing and embrace the knee (right) (shuang fen you lou xi, 雙分右摟膝).

Other Options:

See technique 57, double dividing and embrace the knee (right) (shuang fen you lou xi, 雙分右摟膝).

60. Change Hands and Right Shoulder Stroke (Huan Shou You Kao, 換手右靠)

Movements:

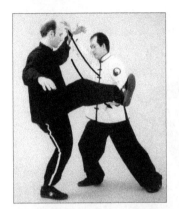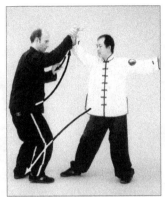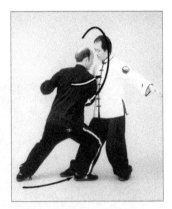

Black pulls his left leg back to the ground and uses his right hand to spread white's right arm to the right. He continues the motion of his right hand by circling it down and to his left to expose white's chest. He immediately steps in with his right leg and strikes white's chest with his shoulder.

Analysis:

This technique is purely for training adhering-sticking and coiling. It is not very practical in a real fight because the large circular motion takes too much time, and your opponent can sense your intention very easily.

Other Options:

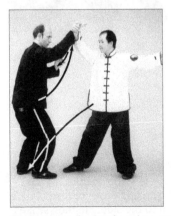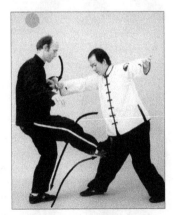

Black can pull white's right wrist down as he puts his left leg down, and simultaneously kick white's groin or stomach with his right foot.

61. Return Right Elbow Stroke (Hui You Kao, 回右靠)

Movements:

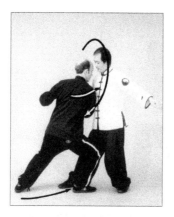 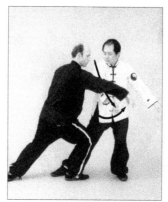

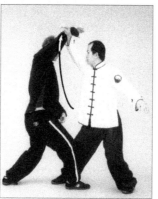 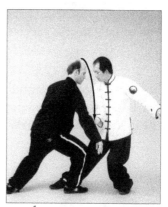

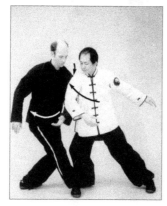

White neutralizes black's strike to his left, then circles his right arm up and down to lead black's arm to the side. He then strikes black's chest with his right shoulder.

Analysis:

See technique 60, change hands and right shoulder stroke (huan shou you kao, 换手右靠).

Other Options:

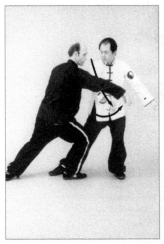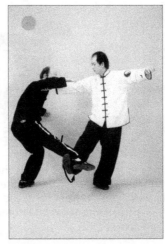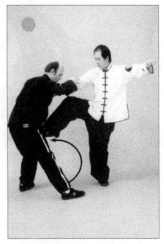

After white has neutralized black's strike, he can use his elbow or shoulder to strike black's chest without circling his arm. Alternatively, he can use his right leg to sweep black's right leg or kick his groin.

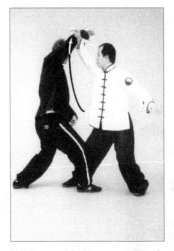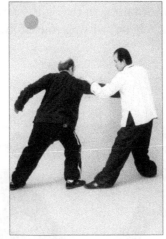

White could also use rollback on black's right arm.

62. Step Forward and Grasp the Sparrow's Tail (Left)
(Shang Bu Zuo Lan Que Wei, 上步左攬雀尾)

Movements:

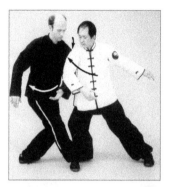 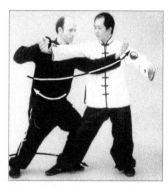

Black twists his body to his right and uses his shoulder and upper arm to neutralize white's shoulder stroke. He then grabs white's right wrist with his right hand and strikes white's chest with his left forearm as he steps his left leg behind white's right leg.

Analysis:

As mentioned in chapter 3, whenever your opponent uses his elbow or shoulder to strike you, you can neutralize the strike either to the right or to the left. Technique 61, return right elbow stroke, is an example of neutralizing to the left while this technique is an example of neutralizing to the right. Remember: to effectively neutralize a short-range strike, you must rely on twisting your body.

Other Options:

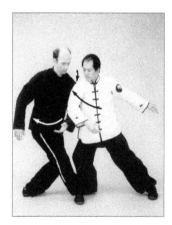 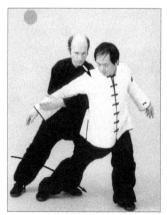

After black has neutralized the strike to his right, he could also strike white's shoulder blade from white's right open door. If black neutralizes the strike to his left, he can follow with a chest attack from white's left open door.

63. Wave Hands in Clouds (Right) (You Yun Shou, 右雲手)

Movements:

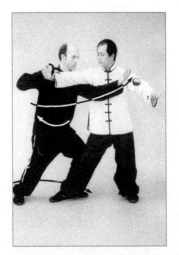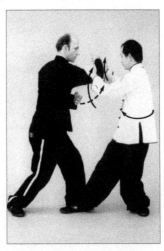

White twists his body to his right, controlling black's right wrist with his right hand, and at the same time uses his left hand to control black's right elbow.

Analysis:

Wave hands in clouds is probably the quickest and most effective way to neutralize black's attack. In order to make the technique effective, white's right hand must grab black's right wrist, and his left hand must control black's elbow to prevent him from using elbow stroke. It is important that white be rooted and stable, otherwise how could he use his body to turn the opponent's body? Right after the neutralization, white must do his next technique immediately because black can easily step his right leg forward and press his chest.

Other Options:

White can use technique 44, strike the tiger, to attack black's temple.

64. Step Forward and Grasp the Sparrow's Tail (Right) (Shang Bu You Lan Que Wei, 上步右攬雀尾)

Movements:

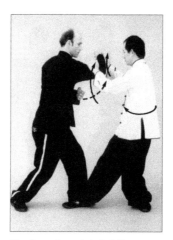 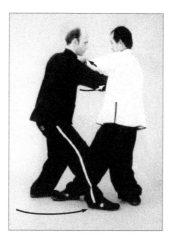

Black grabs white's left wrist with his left hand, steps his right leg forward, and uses his right arm to strike white's body.

Analysis:

Whenever your wrist is grabbed, you lose at least 30 percent of your mobility, and if your elbow is also controlled, you have lost 70 percent of the use of your arm. Therefore, whenever your wrist or elbow is controlled, you should reverse the situation as quickly as possible. Naturally, you would like to control your opponent's wrist and elbow as much as possible so you can put him in a passive situation.

Other Options:

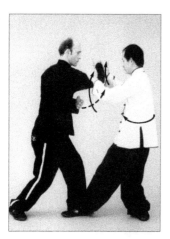 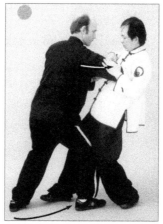

Once black finds his attack has been neutralized to his left, he could immediately step his right leg forward and use his right arm to press white's chest.

65. Wave Hands in Clouds (Left) (Zuo Yun Shou, 右雲手)

Movements:

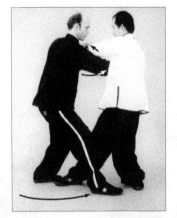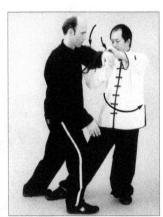

White twists his body to his left while using his left hand to grab black's left wrist and his right hand to control black's elbow.

Analysis:

See technique 63, wave hands in clouds (right) (you yun shou, 右雲手).

Other Options:

White can use technique 44, strike the tiger (right) (you da hu, 右打虎), to strike black's temple.

66. Divide Upward, Press, and Downward Heel Kick (Shang Fen Ji Xia Deng Tui, 上分擠下蹬腿)

Movements:

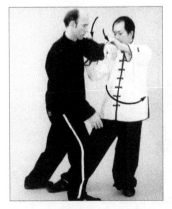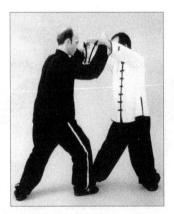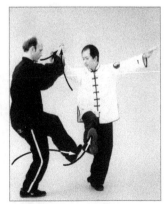

Black uses his right hand to push white's left arm aside and at the same time uses his left hand to open white's right arm. He then uses both hands to press toward white's chest while simultaneously step kicking white's right knee with his left leg.

Analysis:

Kicking is one of the most powerful weapons in taijiquan fighting. Taijiquan specialized in low kicks that are fast and not obvious to the enemy. Very often, a hand technique is used while kicking to distract the opponent's attention. This strategy can be very effective.

Other Options:

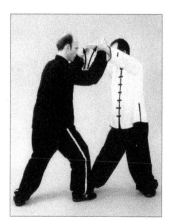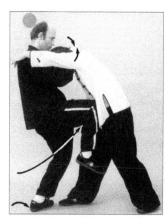

Black can use both hands to grab white's arms or head and then hop kick with his right leg to white's groin or stomach.

67. Low Hook Kick (Xia Gou Tui, 下勾腿)

Movements:

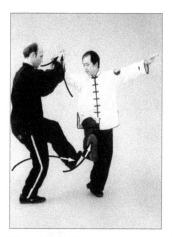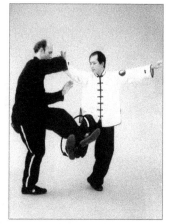

White circles his right arm up to block black's press and lifts his right leg to avoid black's kick, and then immediately uses his right leg to hook black's leg and lift it.

Analysis:

When you fight against an experienced martial artist, you will have little chance of success using your leg to hook his kick. This is because it takes too long to circle your leg, and your opponent can easily sense it. This technique is used here more for training purposes. Usually, the best way to counter a kick to your knee is to withdraw your leg and immediately kick your opponent before he regains his stability.

Other Options:

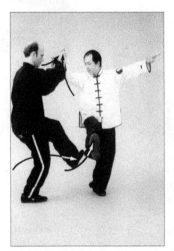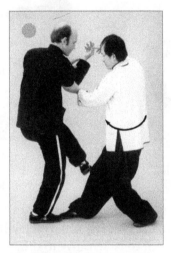

When black attacks with press and a kick, white can use his left hand to grab black's right elbow and pull it to his right while turning his body to his right.

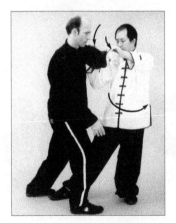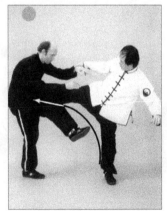

Alternatively, right after white lifts his right leg to avoid black's kick, he can use his right leg to hook backward and kick black's groin or stomach.

68. Turn the Body to Sweep Lotus (Zhuan Shen Bai Lian, 轉身擺蓮)

Movements:

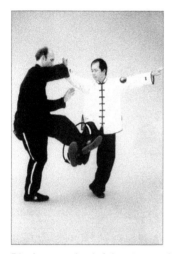 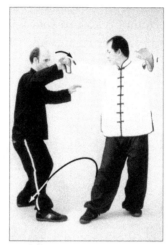 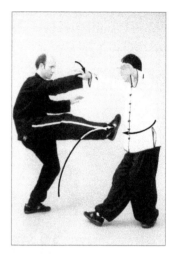

Black raises his left leg to avoid white's hook and steps down while his right hand grabs white's right wrist. He then uses his right leg to sweep kick white's midsection.

Analysis:

In taijiquan, the hooking kick is sometimes used to uproot the opponent's foot. You must train yourself to be sensitive to this.

Other Options:

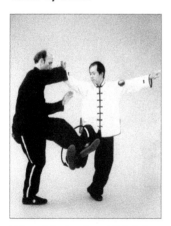 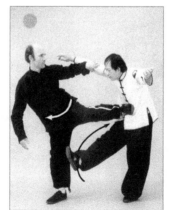 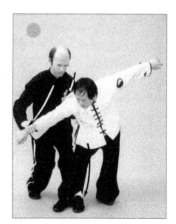

When black raises his left leg to avoid white's hook kick, he can immediately use his heel to back kick white's waist. Alternatively, he can use his right hand to push white's right arm to his right, block white's right leg with his left leg, and rend to destroy his stability.

69. Left Elbow Stroke (Zuo Kao, 左靠)

Movements:

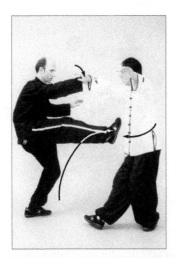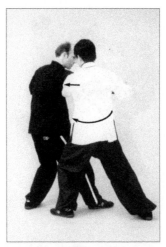

White twists his body to his right and presses his right hand down. He then steps his left leg behind black's right leg and uses his left elbow to strike black under his armpit.

Analysis:

White's best move in this situation is to turn to the right and pull his right hand down. This not only nullifies the kick, but it also sets black up in a bad situation.

Other Options:

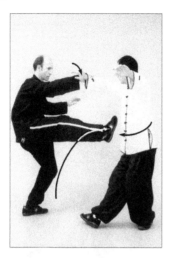 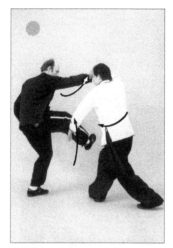

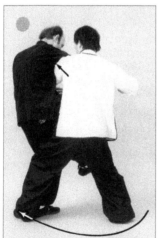 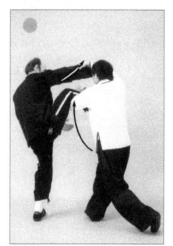

White can push black's right hand to black's left to rend, and at the same time step his left leg forward to bounce black away with a shoulder stroke. Alternatively, while he is turning to his right and pulling his right hand down, he can use his left arm to scoop up black's right leg and knock him off balance.

70. Hook Hand and Snake Creeps Down (Diao Shou She Shen Xia Shi, 刁手蛇身下势)

Movements:

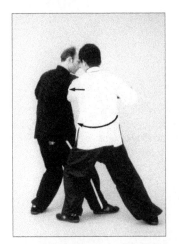 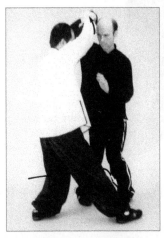 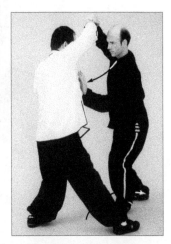

In order to get out of this awkward position, black uses his right hand to grab white's right wrist and pull it to his right. As he is doing this, he steps his left leg opposite white's right open door and then strikes white's chest with his left palm.

Analysis:

This is a good move for black, but he should be aware of one important thing: while he is readjusting his steps, he is very vulnerable, and white can take this opportunity to strike him.

Other Options:

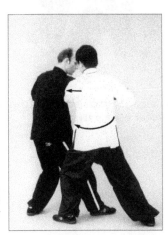 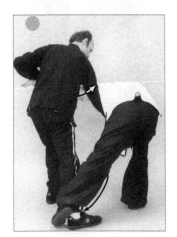

Black can use strike the tiger to attack white's temple as before. Alternatively, black could sweep his right leg backward to destroy white's left root.

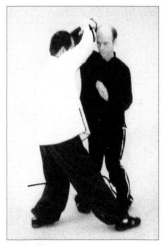

When black is changing his steps, white can take the opportunity to press his right hand down and press black's chest to bounce him away.

71. Diagonal Flying (Right) (You Xie Fei Shi, 右斜飛勢)

Movements:

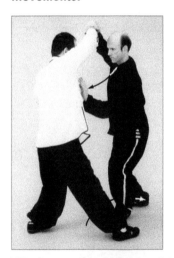 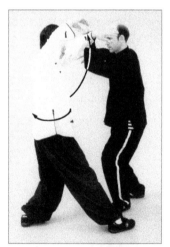 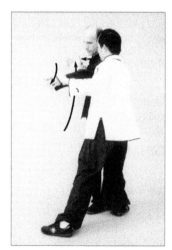

White intercepts upward with his left arm, grabs black's left wrist, and at the same time uses his right arm to execute wardoff under black's armpit.

Analysis:

The best solution for white is to use his right hand to pull down and to black's left. However, when black lifts his right hand and prepares to strike, white has a short time in which he may use his left hand to intercept the strike.

Other Options:

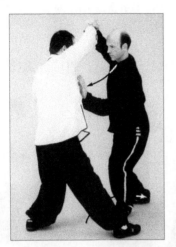 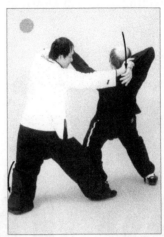

When white uses his left hand to intercept black's strike, white can grab black's right wrist and readjust his steps behind black's body and pull him down from the rear.

72. Strike the Tiger (Left) (Zuo Da Hu, 左打虎)

Movements:

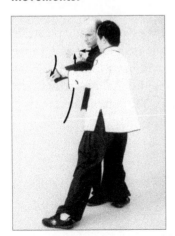 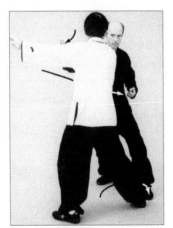 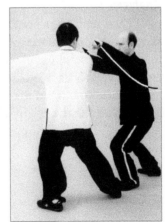

Black uses his right hand to stop white's wardoff, pulls his left hand back as he pushes his right hand forward, and finally strikes white's temple with his left fist.

Analysis:

See technique 6, strike the tiger (right) (you da hu, 右打虎).

Other Options:

See technique 6, strike the tiger (right) (you da hu, 右打虎).

73. Double Dividing and Push Down (Shuang Fen Xia An, 雙分下按)

Movements:

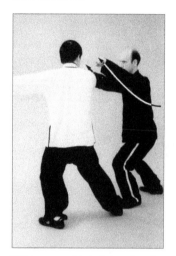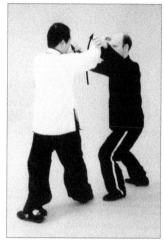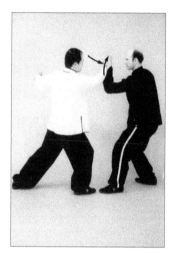

White uses his left hand to free his right hand and at the same time uses his right hand to intercept black's strike. He then uses his right palm to strike black's face or chest.

Analysis:

When both your hands are on the inside of your opponent's hands, and you strike downward or to the face, your power will be limited unless you are good in short-range jing such as inch jing or centimeter jing. In a real fight, you will most likely attack the enemy's eyes, because you will not need too much power to injure them. Alternatively, you can use your hand to reach the enemy's throat and grasp it. Very often, this attack is a fake to attract the enemy's attention.

Other Options:

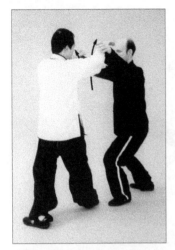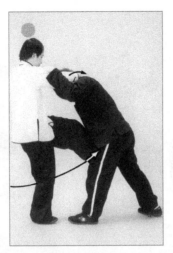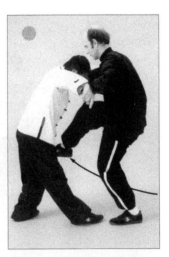

White can use his right hand to hook and press down black's neck and use his left leg to kick black's groin. When black finds that his strike has been neutralized, he can use his right leg to kick white's groin or stomach.

74. Step Back and Repulse Monkey (Dao Nian Hou, 倒攆猴)

Movements:

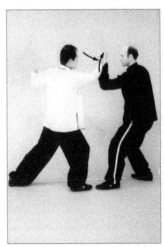

In order to avoid the face strike, black simply sits back and uses his left hand to lead white's strike to the side and then down.

Analysis:

Because black's hand is adhering and sticking with white's right hand, black can easily sense white's intention. He will then sit back to give himself more time and lead white's strike into emptiness.

Other Options:

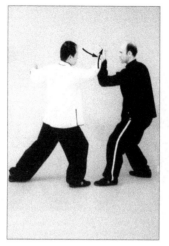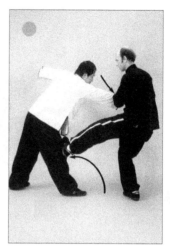

When black sits back, he can use his left leg to kick white's knee.

75. Left Push (Zuo An, 左按)

Movements:

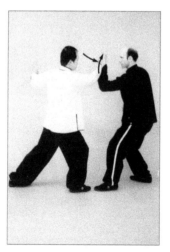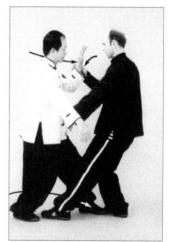

When white finds his right hand has been neutralized to the side and down, he continues his attack by stepping his left leg forward and striking black's face with his left hand.

Analysis:

It is usually necessary to use more than one strike to get your opponent. Your opponent is usually calm enough to escape from your first attack, but if you continue to attack rapidly, you will usually get him with the second or third attack unless he is expert.

Other Options:

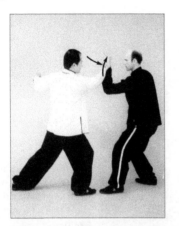
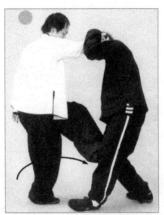

When white finds his right hand neutralized, he can use his left leg to sweep kick black's knee.

76. Step Back and Repulse Monkey (Dao Nian Hou, 倒攆猴)

Movements:

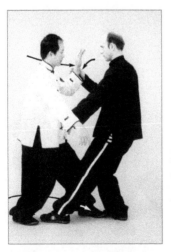
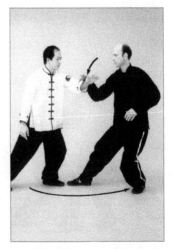

Black uses his right hand to cover white's strike, and at the same time steps back to yield.

Analysis:

See technique 74, step back and repulse monkey (dao nian hou, 倒攆猴).

Other Options:

See technique 74, step back and repulse monkey (dao nian hou, 倒攆猴).

77. Right Push (You An, 右按)

Movements:

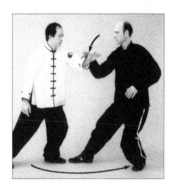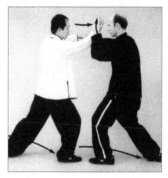

When black neutralizes white's left-hand strike, white steps his right leg forward and use his right palm to strike black's face again.

Analysis:

See technique 75, left push (zuo an, 左按).

Other Options:

See technique 75, left push (zuo an, 左按).

78. Repulse Monkey (Dao Nian Hou, 倒攆猴)

Movements:

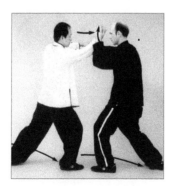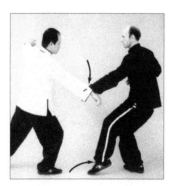

Black again uses his left hand to cover down white's right-hand strike, and this time pulls his left leg back into a false stance.

Analysis:

See technique 74, step back and repulse monkey (dao nian hou, 倒攆猴).

Other Options:

Because black's left leg is empty, he can use it for a quick kick to white's right knee.

79. Right Palm Strike (You Zhang Pai, 右掌拍)

Movements:

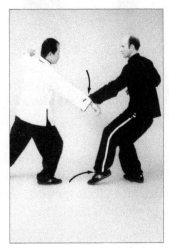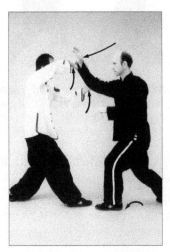

This time, after black has neutralize white's right-hand strike, black will not allow white the opportunity to strike him again. Instead, he steps his left leg forward and strikes white's face with his right palm.

Analysis:

When black strikes with his right hand while his left leg is forward, he has set up for a kick with his right leg to white's stomach or groin.

Other Options:

Immediately after his right palm strike to white's face, black can use his right leg to kick.

80. Step Forward to Seven Stars (Shang Bu Qi Xing, 上步七星)

Movements:

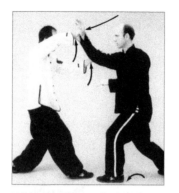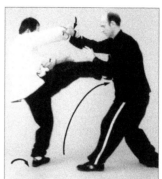

White uses his right hand to intercept black's attack while his left hand controls black's elbow. He then hops up and uses his right leg to kick black's groin or stomach.

Analysis:

In the last technique, when black attacked with his right hand while his left leg was forward, he was in a good position to kick with his rear leg. Here, white can also use his rear leg to kick. In principle, the best way to defend against someone who strikes with one hand when the opposite leg is forward is to block the attacking hand to the other side. This will prevent his kicking from the rear leg.

Other Options:

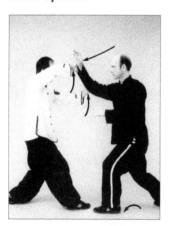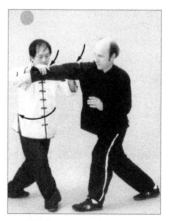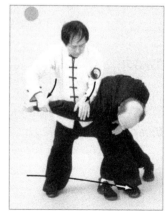

After white blocks black's right-hand strike upward, white can also use both hands to twist black's right hand to black's left, and step his left leg behind black's left leg to make him fall.

81. Pick Up Needle from Sea Bottom (Hai Di Zhen, 海底針)

Movements:

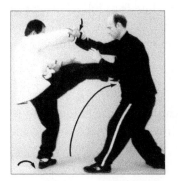 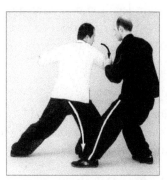

In order to stop white's kick, black uses his right hand to grab white's right hand and pull it down.

Analysis:

As mentioned before, the best strategy for stopping a kick is to pull the opponent's arm down. This will also destroy his balance. Naturally, this only works when you are able to grab your opponent's wrist or arm.

Other Options:

Black can pull to his right and use his left arm to scoop up white's right leg.

82. Fan Back (Shan Tong Bei, 扇通背)

Movements:

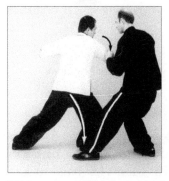 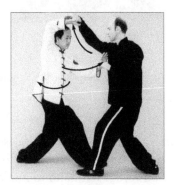

White twists his body to his right and raises his right arm, and uses his left hand to strike black under the armpit.

Analysis:

In fact, this is a difficult and perhaps even dangerous technique. When white pulls his arm up, if black can easily free his hand, he can use that opportunity to kick white's groin with his right leg. The best strategy for white is to follow black's pull and readjust his body to black's right open door to reverse the situation. As white does this, he should not step too close to black, otherwise black can use the opportunity to press or push him and make him lose balance.

Other Options:

When white raises his right arm, black can follow the motion and pull white's right hand to white's left. This will stop white's left-hand strike. He should immediately push forward to bounce white off balance.

83. Pluck Right (You Cai, 右採)

Movements:

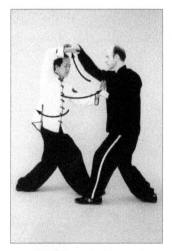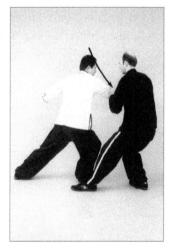

Again, black plucks white's right wrist and pulls it down.

Analysis:

The best strategy against white's strike is to pull his right hand down as shown in this technique. However, sometimes you will find that you do not have enough time to do this. In this case, use your left hand to intercept white's left-hand strike.

Other Options:

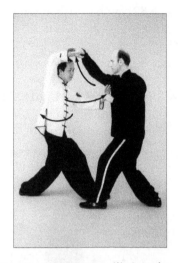

When white raises up his right hand, black can use this opportunity to kick white's groin with his right leg. Because a leg is longer than an arm, black does not have to worry too much about white's left-hand strike.

84. Draw the Bow and Shoot the Tiger (Wan Gong She Hu, 彎弓射虎)

Movements:

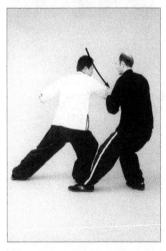 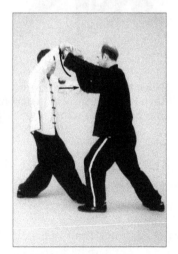

White again raises up his right arm and at the same time intends to use his left fist to strike black under the armpit.

Analysis:

See technique 82, fan back (shan tong bei, 扇通背).

Other Options:

See technique 82, fan back (shan tong bei, 扇通背).

85. Neutralize Up and Press Forward (Xia Hua Ping Ji, 下化平擠)

Movements:

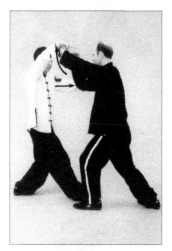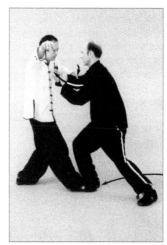

When black senses white's hand rising, he uses both hands to open white's arms. He then immediately steps forward and uses both hands to press white's chest.

Analysis:

As explained in technique 82, fan back, the best strategy for black to use against white's pull up is to let go and at the same time use his right leg to kick white's groin.

Other Options:

See technique 83, pluck right (you cai, 右採).

86. Punch under the Elbow (Zhou Di Kan Chui, 肘底看捶)

Movements:

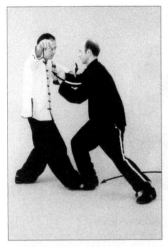 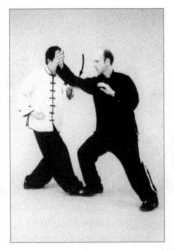 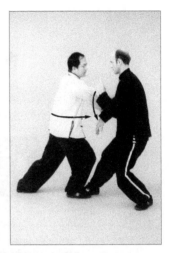

White uses his left hand to push black's right elbow to his right, and then uses his right fist to punch black under the armpit.

Analysis:

To defend against a press, you should turn your body to the side, and if possible, control the opponent's elbow to lead the press sideward.

Other Options:

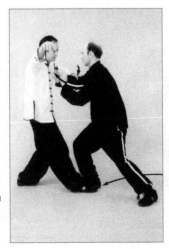

White can twist his body to his left and use his right upper arm to neutralize the press. He can then press or strike black from black's left open door.

87. Cross Hands (Shi Zi Shou, 十字手)

Movements:

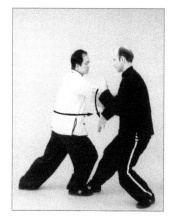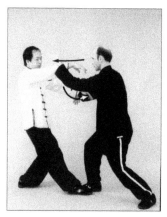

Black moves his right arm down while he is sitting back to lead white's punch to the side. Black then uses his left hand to strike white's face.

Analysis:

You should understand that sometimes your opponent will grab your right elbow and will not allow you to pull it back and use it to block the punch. In this case, you should rotate your body to your right and use your left hand to protect your chest.

Other Options:

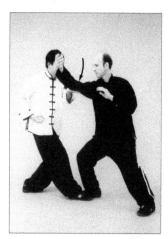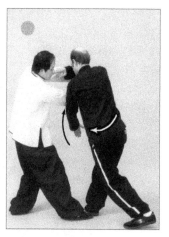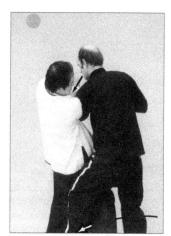

Black can turn his body to his right and use his left arm to intercept white's punch. Black can then step his left leg forward and press white's chest.

88. Embrace Tiger and Return to the Mountain (Bao Hu Gui Shan, 抱虎歸山)

Movements:

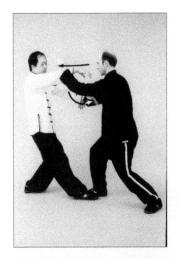 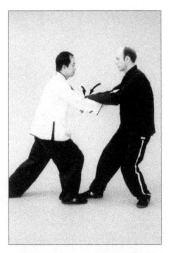

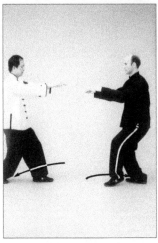 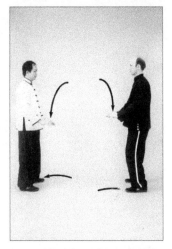

White raises his right hand to intercept black's strike and uses his left hand to lead black's right hand to the side. White then pushes both hands forward to black's chest. When black senses white's push, he immediately presses both hands down to neutralize it. Finally, both white and black step backward to end the fighting set.

Chapter 5: Taijiquan Fighting Strategy

5-1. Introduction

It is not unusual for martial artists who have practiced for many years to still get beaten up by people who have had little or no actual martial training. For example, a martial artist who has won trophies for tournament sparring may end up on the ground in a street fight because he trained only for tournaments and emphasized techniques that gain points, rather than techniques that are effective for self-defense. Many martial artists emphasize offensive training and neglect defensive training. If you train for tournaments where attacks to the face and groin are illegal, you will tend to leave them unguarded and not develop effective ways of protecting them. Because these areas are favorite targets for street fighters, you may be training yourself to lose fights.

There is another very important factor that could make a tournament fighter become a dead street fighter, and that is the factor of bravery and mental preparation. A tournament fight is a game and not a real, deadly fight. Both you and your opponent control your power and avoid attacking vital areas. However, losing a fight in the street may mean losing your life. Of course, it cannot be denied that the more sparring experience you have, the more confidence and preparation you will have. However, if your practice fights with your friends or tournament competitors do not have the same sense or feeling of a street fight, you run the risk in a street fight of losing the ability to fight effectively. You may be very good defending against a rubber knife, but how good are you against a real one?

The same thing can also happen to a gongfu fighter even if he has built the habit of protecting the vital areas. In Chinese martial society, there is a saying: "First, bravery; second, power; and third, gongfu" (Yi dan, er li, san gongfu, 一膽、二力、三功夫). This means that in a real fight, bravery is the first requirement for success. If a person is brave and has a strong spirit, then even if he does not have any gongfu experience, he can still have a good chance of beating a scared martial artist.

It is unfortunately fairly common for people who have developed a high degree of skill in pushing-hands contests to be unable to defend themselves against external-style martial artists or street fighters. This has come about because in the last fifty years the real taijiquan fighting has been ignored. Pushing hands, which is a friendly and harmless way to compete, has been used as a standard for judging taijiquan fighting ability. Unfortunately, in a real fight, nobody will cross hands with you and play pushing hands. Instead, an adversary will punch or kick you with as much speed and power as possible. If you do not know how to react, if you have not learned how to adhere-connect and then stick-follow, you will become a victim of his power. Therefore, in order to become a real taijiquan martial artist, you must learn how to handle a quick and powerful attack such as a punch or kick. You must remember that in a real fight, there is no time for you to think and then react—everything must be a natural reaction. This means you must train realistically.

This chapter will focus on the fighting techniques and strategy that have been neglected by taijiquan for the past fifty years. The second section will discuss various considerations that arise in a fight. The third section will discuss how taijiquan fighters connect in a fight, and the fourth section will discuss timing. The fifth section will discuss how jing is used in a fight, and the sixth section will present translations of several poems and songs that pertain to fighting strategy.

5-2. About a Real Fight

Before the Fight

Before you get into a fight, you must first ask yourself a few things: Is this fight necessary? What is my motivation in this fight? What are my chances of winning? What will the consequences be?

1. Knowing Your Purpose and Motivation in Fighting

I remember something my White Crane master told me repeatedly. He said, "If a person asks for a fight because his dignity is hurt, then his morality is poor. If you accept the fight, then your morality is no higher than his. However, if you can be humble and bow, then your morality is higher than his. It takes a lot of courage to do this. Humility is not the behavior of a coward; on the contrary, it is the expression of courage, wisdom, calm, and tolerance. If you fight just to protect your dignity, then the fight is not worthy."

On the other hand, if you are forced to fight to protect your life or to protect your family or a friend, then you should fight bravely. Under such circumstances, nobody would blame you. Because you are motivated by a good purpose, you will not hesitate or be afraid to accept the fight.

You should know one thing: if you ask for a fight because your dignity is hurt, then you are not a hero. You are just a coward because you behave exactly like a coward, asking for more respect and dignity. Remember: a person must despise himself first before people will despise him. Therefore, if you can avoid a fight, you should.

If your fight is just sparring with a friend or in a competition, then both you and your opponent must control your tempers. It is easy for one side to lose his temper and start a real fight. If you find the opponent has a bad temper and cannot control himself, then you should avoid the fight. Remember that anything can happen in a fight—so be prepared.

2. Knowing the Consequences of a Fight

Even if you have a good reason to accept a fight, you must also consider the consequences of the fight. You may feel satisfied after you have won the fight, but have you considered the possibility that the opponent will try to take revenge? Is it possible that he may come after you with a gun or with a group of his friends? After the fight, will you have to live in fear of his revenge? What have you proved with the fight after all? Are you a coward or a hero? Or are you just a small man like your opponent and other street fighters? Will you earn more respect from this fight or you will make all your real friends leave you? All these questions will have to be considered when you are faced with the possibility of a fight. No one else can decide what is right for you at that time. No one else can take responsibility for your decisions.

3. Knowing Yourself and the Enemy

If you decide that you have a good reason to fight, you must then consider several other things: How good is this enemy? What are my chances of winning? Will my fighting spirit be able to overcome bad circumstances such as a smaller body or limited fighting experience? For example, if you are alone against five opponents, would it be smarter to avoid the fight or even run away? Running is not necessarily a cowardly act. Sometimes it is the best thing to do. Sun Zi's book on fighting strategy concluded that running away is the best strategy.

4. Knowing the Location of the Fight

The last thing you must consider before you start the fight is the location. Is the place big enough to fit your style? If the opponent suddenly uses a concealed knife, could you find a stick or rock for defense? If you cannot win the fight, can you escape easily? For example, if you specialize in kicks, you should not fight on a slippery surface like ice.

Before Contact

Taijiquan is a martial style that specializes in short-range fighting. Most of the techniques are based on and developed from adhering-sticking. Middle-range fighting, which uses a limited amount of kicking, is used but is not commonly seen. Long-range fighting, in which kicking plays a major role, is mostly ignored in taiji. Therefore, if you are a taijiquan fighter and are about to fight, you must know several important things. Do you know how to avoid long-range attacks? How do you approach the opponent safely and move into middle and short range? Do you know how to connect and intercept so you can use your taijiquan techniques? These questions are probably the most important for today's taijiquan martial artists, because these types of training have been neglected for the last fifty years. In this subsection we will briefly discuss the importance of these items, and in the next section we will discuss them more thoroughly.

1. Knowing the Suitable Fighting Distance

Taijiquan specializes in short-range fighting, with middle range second in importance and long range last. You therefore want to stay at short range because it is the most advantageous for you. If your opponent is also in a style that specializes in short-range fighting, such as Crane or Snake styles, your techniques must be higher than your opponent's in order to win the fight. If your opponent is in a style that specializes in long-range fighting, such as Long Fist or Praying Mantis, then you must be aware of what distance is most advantageous for his kicking. For different opponents, the strategy can be completely different. The key to winning a fight is to always maintain the fighting distance that is most advantageous for you.

2. Knowing the Enemy's Fighting Capability

In order to set up your fighting strategy, you must first know your enemy's ability and strategy. Going into a fight blind is dangerous. There are several ways you can discover your opponent's fighting potential and specialties. First, you can judge him pretty well if you know what style he has learned. For example, Long Fist style will be good in long-range kicking techniques. Second, you can use a fake attack to test his awareness, reaction, speed, and spirit. Third, you can often tell a lot about a person from his facial expression. For example, if his face is calm but reactive, and his steps stable and steady, then you know you face a strong opponent.

3. Knowing the Ways of Avoiding an Attack

Once you know the situation for both of you, then you must also know the ways and techniques of avoiding your opponent's attack. We will discuss these techniques and strategy in the next section.

4. Knowing How to Trick the Enemy

You must know how to trick and fake the opponent and create the opportunity for you to move into medium and short range safely and effectively. This will also be discussed in the next section.

5. Knowing How to Connect

Once you have closed the distance to short range, you must know how to intercept and connect to the opponent so that you can use taijiquan techniques. This will be discussed in the next section.

After Contact

Once you have connected with your enemy, you must use several skills that have been developed through long practice of pushing hands. Because they have been discussed in previous chapters, we will just list the important points here to refresh your memory.

1. Knowing the enemy's intention through touch.
2. Knowing how to adhere and stick.
3. Knowing taijiquan techniques and strategy.
4. Knowing the taijiquan jing.

Fighting Attitude

In addition to all of these, you must also develop your fighting spirit and attitude, which are usually the most important factors in winning.

1. Bravery

Bravery is the most important factor in winning a fight. When you are scared, your muscles generate acid, which makes them tremble and feel sore. This greatly lessens your capacity to fight. Therefore, before you fight, you must know why you are fighting, and once you are committed to the fight, you should be straightforward and not hesitate.

2. Confidence

In order to be brave, you must have confidence in your fighting ability. You must know what you are doing and what to expect. A fight without confidence is usually a fight lost. Confidence is built through accumulating fighting experience.

3. Calmness and Firmness

Once you have bravery and confidence, you should then learn to avoid getting excited. An excited mind can be easily fooled. You must remain calm, and your technique and strategy must be firm. Use your calm mind to judge the situation and your firm technique to execute your thoughts.

4. Decisiveness

Once you are committed to a fight, you must be mentally and emotionally prepared to act decisively and win the fight. This usually means hurting the opponent. Beware of unwarranted mercy or concern for the person who is trying to hurt you. If you hesitate in a fight, or "pull your punches," you may give your opponent the opportunity to beat you. Once you are committed to an attack, there is no room for regret or changing your mind. This doesn't mean that you must be brutal or cruel, but it does mean that you must be determined to win and must act decisively.

5. Spirit

In a fight, your spirit must be kept high. This is especially important in taijiquan. When your spirit is raised, your qi will be full and stimulated, and consequently, your jing will be strong. A high spirit will also enhance your bravery.

6. Agility

Your thought, movement, and techniques must be agile. When they are agile they are fast and alive, and your opponent has a harder time figuring out what technique and strategy you are going to use.

7. Liveliness

In a fight, your steps and techniques must be alive. This means you must be aware of the opponent's every movement, and you must respond to his every change. When your steps and techniques are alive, you can skillfully change from insubstantial to substantial and vice versa.

8. Cautiousness

Even if you are brave, you must also be cautious. This is why, when you fight, you need to have a calm mind to judge the situation. Like playing chess, one wrong step might lose the whole fight.

9. Sneakiness

Once you have decided to fight, it is a fight. You must be sneaky and fake out the opponent without being faked out yourself. You must learn how to use techniques that look real but are not and techniques that do not look real but are.

10. Ability to Overwhelm

The ability to overwhelm the opponent is built upon your confidence. As in playing chess, always make your opponent feel that he is passive and under your control. Make him feel when he advances that the distance is becoming longer and longer, and when he retreats that the distance between you is becoming shorter and shorter and his situation ever-more urgent. You are the one controlling the entire fighting situation. You are the master. If you have this feeling, you have already won the fight.

Fighting Moralities

Finally, there is something else that a good taijiquan fighter should have, and that is morality. There are five aspects to morality:

1. Endurance

In order to become a good taijiquan fighter, you must endure the pain other people cannot endure, control the temper other people cannot control, and be humble when other people cannot be humble. Endurance is the key to success. If you can endure, then you will be patient and perseverant, and you will be able to enter the deeper level of taiji meditation and qi circulation.

2. Tolerance

In order to become a wise taijiquan master, you must be able to tolerate the emotion that other people cannot tolerate and endure the anguish that other people cannot endure.

3. Humanity

In order to become a great and kind master, you must love what other people cannot love. You must help those whom other people aren't willing to help. You must concern yourself with the events with which other people do not concern themselves. You must respect your parents and elders and also love other people's parents and elders. You must love your own children as well as other people's children.

4. Forgiveness

You must forgive the person other people cannot forgive. As you understand your point of view, so should you also understand the opponent's point of view. When you can see both sides, it is easier to forgive and live in happiness. Even though you have won the battle, you should be humble enough to apologize and ask for forgiveness. Very often, this will turn your enemy into your friend and put an end to hate and further fighting. When you injure your opponent, you should help him as much as possible after the fight.

5. Peace

You must always have a peaceful mind. Fighting is the last solution. When you have a peaceful mind, you have fewer enemies, and you can judge good and bad more clearly. A peaceful mind lets you be happy and appreciate your life.

5-3. How to Connect in Taijiquan Fighting

Many taiji martial artists have had difficulty in street fights, even though they have practiced pushing hands and the two-person set for many years. There are several reasons for this. First, most people in taijiquan have not had any real sparring experience. Most taijiquan practice today is limited to the techniques used after connecting with the enemy. A real fight, however, will not usually start out with your hands in contact with the opponent's; instead, he will attack you with fast punches and kicks. If you do not have experience in connecting, you will surely fall victim to a practical street fighter. Therefore, in order to be able to use your taijiquan techniques in a real fight, you must learn how to connect.

A second reason why taijiquan people sometimes have difficulty in fights is that even those who have learned how to connect have not always built up the habit of accessing the open doors. Even if you have fast reactions and can intercept and connect to a punch, if you do not use the right position and footwork, you might give your opponent the opportunity to attack you. Therefore, when you learn how to connect, you must also learn how to position yourself. A third reason is that taijiquan martial artists frequently ignore the kicking techniques. Because kicking techniques are not heavily emphasized in the sequence, many people think kicking techniques are not particularly useful. However, low kicks are fast and very effective, and they are actually an important part of taijiquan fighting. If you do not know how to coordinate your kicking techniques with your hands, your fighting capability will be significantly reduced.

The following section will introduce several training methods. I hope they will give you some ideas on how to start learning how to connect.

How to React

The most important thing in a fight is reaction. When someone punches at you, you must react quickly and naturally. Because in that situation you will not have time to think, you need to have built up your natural intercepting ability. Once you have intercepted, then you can connect. There are many ways of training your reactions in both external and internal styles. Because taijiquan emphasizes connecting and sticking, its reaction training must emphasize coiling and controlling instead of just blocking and intercepting. Before we discuss how to step and set up your position, we would first like to introduce exercises for reacting to and connecting with an attack. Because your eyes are first to sense the opponent's attack, it is important to train the eyes to develop your reaction speed. This exercise will also train you to not blink, as well as develop your ability to spot attacks as they form and start. In order to avoid injury, you and your partner should only attack the forehead. You should practice until you can intercept and connect naturally without blinking or closing your eyes, even when the attack is very fast and sudden. Naturally, when you train, you must start slowly and only speed up as your skill increases.

Drill 1

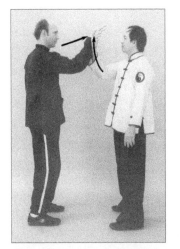 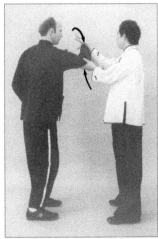

Black tries to touch white's forehead with his right hand, and white lifts his right forearm to intercept. When the right hand connects, white uses his left hand to touch black's elbow while his right hand coils down.

When your arm comes from in front of your body and deflects the opponent's arm to the outside, it is called repelling. If your partner withdraws suddenly right after you have intercepted, but before you could stick and coil, follow his withdrawal and attack his forehead. The training is mutual. However, in the beginning, it is important to train with one side only attacking and the other only defending, until both persons can intercept and connect naturally.

Drill 2

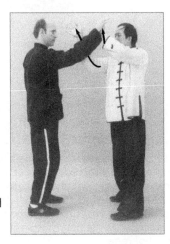 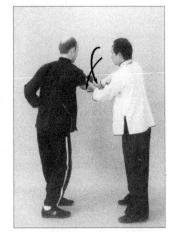

Black tries to touch white's forehead with his right hand. White uses his right forearm and left hand to intercept the attack. White then circles both hands down and to the side, with his right hand controlling black's forearm and his left hand on his elbow. This technique is usually called cover.

Drill 3

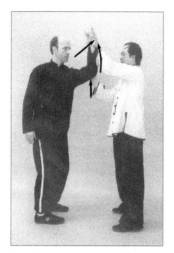 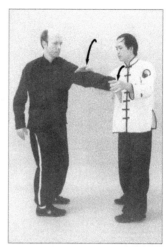

Black uses his left hand to touch white's forehead. White uses his left hand to repel intercept black's forearm while his right hand controls black's elbow. Black then circles down and uses his left hand to control white's wrist while his right hand controls white's elbow.

Drill 4

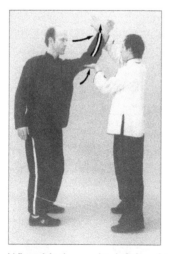 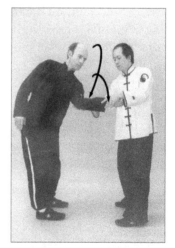

When black uses his left hand to touch white's forehead, white uses his right hand to repel intercept and touches black's elbow with his left hand. After white intercepts, he continues the circular motion downward to control black's wrist and elbow. In this attack, if white uses his left hand to intercept black's attack, it is similar to the first motion in drill 2 and is called cover instead of repel.

Once you have mastered the above drills and can defend yourself easily through intercepting, connecting, and coiling, you should then start attacking and defending two spots—the forehead and chest—and see if you can still react naturally. Once you can react naturally, you should next learn how to step.

How to Step

Even if you learn from these drills how to react naturally to an attack, your defense is still lacking because you have not yet learned how to move into the best position for the next move, and your opponent may still be active and in a position to attack you further. You must therefore know how to step and put your enemy into a passive position right after you connect. This section will offer you some examples of stepping for this purpose.

Drill 1

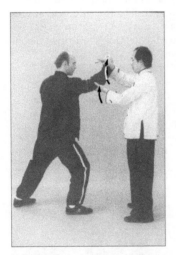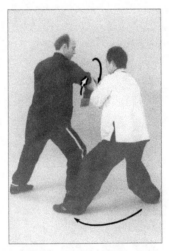

When black throws a right punch to white's upper body, white uses both hands to connect. White then coils both hands down to control black's right arm and at the same time steps in with his left leg to access black's right open door.

Drill 2

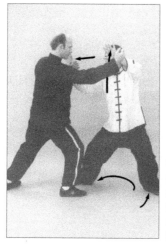

When black uses his right hand to punch white's chest, white uses his left hand to intercept and repel to the side, and at the same time he repositions himself to access black's left open door.

Drill 3

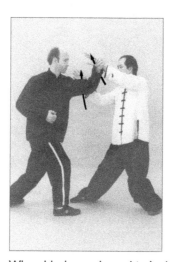 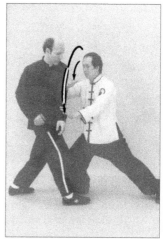

When black punches white's chest with his left hand while his right leg is forward, white uses both hands to intercept and connect, and at the same time repositions himself to access black's left open door. In order to prevent black from kicking with his left leg, black immediately coils both his hands down to put black in an awkward position.

Drill 4

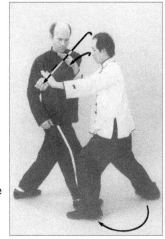

In drill 3, after white connects, he can also step his left leg to the outside of black's right leg, and press with both hands to put black in an awkward position.

Defense against Kicks

Taijiquan emphasizes short-range fighting, so low kicks are used more often than middle-level and high kicks. Low kicks are usually powerful and fast, and they can be very hard to see and react to. It is very important for a taijiquan fighter to connect and stick with the opponent, because this gives him the chance to sense and react to a kick. Because he is in contact, he will be able to easily push or pull the opponent's upper body down to upset his balance and stop the kick. You usually do not need much time to train yourself to react this way to low kicks, because whenever anyone kicks, he must move his upper body first. Because a taijiquan fighter is in contact with the opponent and has been trained by pushing hands to sense motion, he should not have a great deal of difficulty sensing low kicks. It is necessary, however, to learn to distinguish the different kinds of kicks and to learn to stop them before they get started.

If a taijiquan player is fighting against a martial artist of a different style, the fight may not start at short range, so he must know how to defend against middle- and long-range kicks. Usually, you can see middle- and long-range kicks coming, and you have more time to react. However, such kicks can still be fast and very powerful. Because you are not in contact with the opponent, you will not be able to sense the kicks by touch, so visual reaction and stepping become very important. The best strategy against a powerful kick is not to block, because you may injure yourself. Instead, you should move to avoid the attack and access the opponent's open door. Naturally, accessing the opponent's open door without blocking is difficult and takes a great deal of training.

Before trying to access the opponent's open door without blocking the kick, you should first master neutralizing the kick and accessing the open door at the same time. Here are two examples of the many exercises that are commonly used for training.

Drill 1

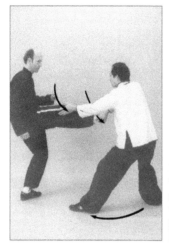

Black kicks with his right leg to white's groin or stomach. White slides both of his feet to the side to reposition himself and at the same time uses both hands to lead the kick to his right.

Drill 2

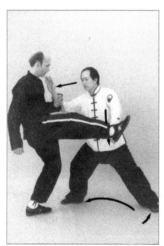

White could reposition himself to black's left empty door and at the same time use his left hand to lead the kick to his left.

Faking

When your opponent is cautious and does not attack first, it is often difficult to find an opportunity to connect. When this happens, you simply play an active role and attack first. Naturally, you know this attack will most likely be blocked, but this is exactly what you want, for you will then have the opportunity to connect to his block.

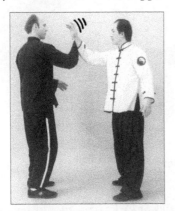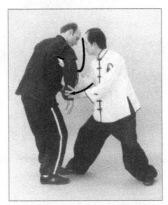

Use your right hand to attack your opponent's eyes. He has to intercept your attack, and when he does, you immediately connect, stick, and coil. You now have the chance to create an opportunity for a real attack. For example, you can coil down and attack his armpit.

Low Kicks

Low kicks are fast and powerful and are commonly used in taijiquan fighting, so you must know how to use them. We will give you four examples.

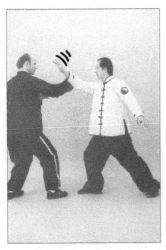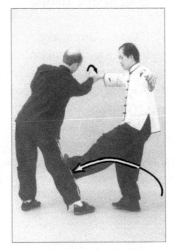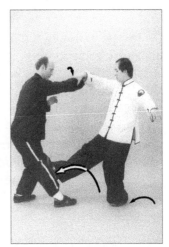

Right after you connect after faking an attack or intercepting one, immediately control the opponent's wrist and use either leg to step kick his knee.

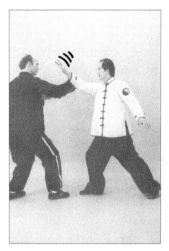 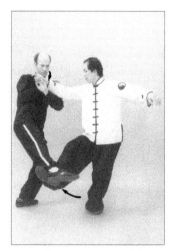 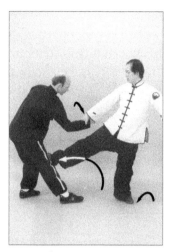

After contact, you could use your right leg to sweep his right leg or stamp kick his right knee.

In order to learn more options and varieties of kicks, you should review the kicking jing in chapter 3 of the book *Tai Chi Chuan Martial Power: Advanced Yang Style*, 3rd edition, from YMAA Publication Center.

Because of the limitations of space, this section can offer you only ideas and guidelines for training. There are many other ways of training that you can use to continue your practice. Remember: the art of taijiquan is not really alive until you know how to use it, and how much you learn is determined by your effort and imagination.

5-4. Attack Timing

In a fight, timing is probably the most important factor in determining if your techniques are going to work. The right timing can not only allow you to avoid the enemy's attack, but it also gives you the chance to successfully attack your enemy. You can learn all the good techniques from the sequence and know how to apply them, but if you do not practice pushing hands, the fighting set, and free fighting, you will never be able to use your techniques in a real fight. In order to train timing, you must build your natural reaction beyond what you think is possible. If you develop your natural reactions correctly, you will gradually build up a natural understanding of attack and defensive timing as you accumulate experience. Below we will present a song (adage) that discusses and analyzes attack timing. We hope this song will give you a fairly good idea of timing in a fight.

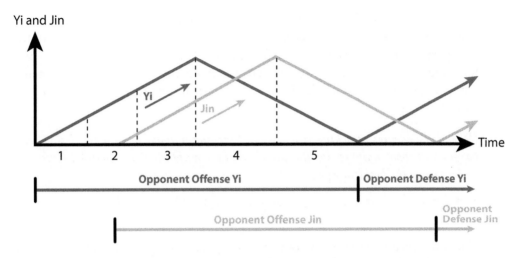

Generally speaking, when your enemy intends to attack you, he must generate his attacking yi first. His qi is also generated at this time, but it does not yet show in his postures. A high-level martial artist will be able to sense his opponent's intention through the expression on his face or even by sensing his qi. When the opponent's yi has grown to a certain level, his jing will start to grow. When his yi has reached the maximum, his jing will still be growing. When his jing has reached its maximum, his yi has usually started to withdraw, which causes his jing to stop and start to withdraw as well. Remember: yi comes first, then qi. This qi will then support the jing so that it reaches its maximum. Before jing reaches its maximum, the yi has already been there. When jing reaches its maximum, yi has already started to withdraw. If you can analyze the timing following this rule, you will be able to catch the meaning of the following song.

Attack Timing Strategy 攻時略
Dr. Yang, Jwing-Ming 楊俊敏

> *[When] enemy's attacking yi is forming and his posture has not yet shown, I suddenly attack and disturb his yi and stop the forming of his posture. [This] is reaching "enlightenment." [This timing] is the best among the best strategies.*

> 敵擊意已孕， 而勢未現， 我驟然反攻以亂其意， 挫其勢之孕形， 是為通乎神明，
> 乃為上上策。

Remember: yi is always ahead of qi, and where the yi is, there is also the qi. When you have developed your qi, you can use it to support your jing as you express it through your posture. Therefore, when you sense the enemy's qi, it means that his yi is forming, and his qi is not yet strong enough to support jing. If you attack just when you sense his intention and qi, you can disturb the forming of his yi and qi and put him into a passive, disadvantageous situation. It takes a great deal of experience to sense the opponent's intention. This is one of the timings used for "cold jing" (*leng jing*, 冷勁). When you reach this stage, you have reached "enlightenment." Naturally, this is the best among the best timings in attacking the enemy.

[When] the enemy's attacking yi shows, and his jing is about to emit but hasn't yet, I borrow this opportunity to stop [his attack] and interrupt his yi and posture. [It is] normally among the best strategies.

敵擊意己現，　而勁將出未出，　我借此機，　阻其意、其勢，　乃上平策。

When the enemy's yi is about complete, his qi has been generated and is ready to support jing. If I take this time to interrupt his yi and stop his jing, the jing he generated will bounce back to him. Because his yi is almost complete, it is totally concentrated on attacking, and he will not be able to instantly stop his attacking yi and withdraw his qi and jing. His jing will therefore be bounced back. This is the first timing of borrowing jing.

[When] the enemy's attacking yi is completed and jing has been emitted, I must first stop his [attacking] posture [and] then counterattack. [This is] the most common strategy.

敵攻意己成，　勢亦已發，　我必先阻其勢而反擊，　乃平策。

When the enemy's yi is completed and his jing is emitted, I must block or avoid his attack first, and then counterattack. This timing is a common one that most of the martial artists can do.

[When] the enemy's attacking yi is weakening and his attacking posture is strongest, I borrow his jing and reverse [the situation] to check his posture. [This is] the difficult one of the best strategies.

敵攻意漸踬，　攻勢正盛，　我借其勁而反挫其勢，　是為上難策。

When the enemy's jing has reached its maximum, his attacking yi will be weakening. However, at this time, his jing will be the strongest. If I know how to borrow his jing at this moment, I will be able to bounce him away. This is the more difficult level of borrowing jing.

[When] the enemy's attacking yi is ended and his defensive yi is about to generate, his posture moves back for defense, I borrow this opportunity and follow his posture and attack. [It is] the easiest one of the best strategies.

敵攻意已盡，守意將生，勢正回守，我借此機而反攻，是為上易策。

When the enemy's attacking yi is ended and his yi is about to withdraw, you should take this opportunity and attack in along his extended limb before he withdraws it. When his yi is about to withdraw, his defensive capability is weak, and vital areas are exposed because his arm is extended. If you take this moment to attack just as he is starting to withdraw, you will certainly get him unless he is very good in sticking hands.

5-5. Jing in a Fight

It is not uncommon for people to understand the deeper theory of jing but not be able to use it. It cannot be denied that theory is the foundation of the application of jing. However, if you do not know the tricks and secrets of training it, you will waste a lot of time in experimentation and research before you develop the ability to use it effectively.

As a matter of fact, the secret of jing is in your breath. Through your breathing you control and lead the qi in and out. Your breathing determines whether the qi is long or short, strong or weak, and it is your breathing that reveals if your qi is smooth or stagnant. In Chinese martial society, it is common to observe a person's breathing to judge the smoothness and strength of his qi and jing. Therefore, when you begin training, you should practice your breathing first. The breathing must be smooth and round, full and strong. You must be able to coordinate your breathing with your fighting strategy. Breathing is like a mirror for qi—you can look at your breathing to see what your qi is doing. This is why Chinese martial artists usually use the word "qi" to represent both air and internal energy.

Once your breathing becomes natural and united with your qi, you should transfer your yi to your opponent. When you generate yi, your breathing and qi naturally follow, and so your qi can automatically support your jing. Remember: the final goal is that your yi is on your enemy, not on your breathing. When it is on your breathing, you are stagnant. When it is on your opponent, you can be natural and alive.

You should now understand that your breathing is of greatest importance in both pushing hands and fighting. Breathing follows your strategy, but it governs your qi and jing, so you must understand how to control your breathing in a fight.

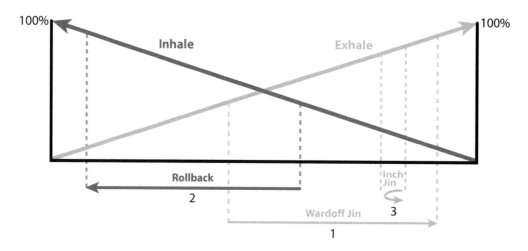

Coordination of Breathing and Jin

In principle, when you breathe in a fight, you should never inhale or exhale to the limit. Of course, it cannot be denied that the fuller your inhalation and exhalation, the more qi you will generate. However, if you inhale and exhale to the maximum, you will have difficulty changing your strategy. Furthermore, such maximum breathing makes your qi stagnant, which causes your jing to be dull and dead. In the illustration above, the exhalation is to the right and the inhalation is to the left. The area under the inhalation or exhalation line is the size of your breath and the jing you have generated. When you are in a fight, your breathing should be in the center. Remember: the longer your breathing, the stronger your qi will be (except for the extreme breathing, which should be avoided). In the diagram, area 1 under the exhale line shows the exhalation and the jing for wardoff as you emit jing. Area 2 under the inhale line represents the inhalation and defensive jing of rollback. Either jing can be long or short, strong or more restrained. Area 3 shows the jing of the shortest jing such as inch jing and centimeter jing, where you inhale and exhale quickly. Naturally, the power will not be as strong as other jing.

Hopefully this discussion has helped you gain some idea of the secret of jing. I would like to conclude with a poem.

The Secret of Jing 勁訣篇
Dr. Yang, Jwing-Ming 楊俊敏

The secret of jing is in the qi, the circulation of qi is in the breath. Qi and the breath's fast and slow determine jing's long and short; full or deficient gauge jing's strong and weak.

勁之訣在氣，氣之行決於息。氣息之快緩，定勁之長短、沛謙，測勁之猛蹶。

Modulate breath properly, qi will be smooth and exchangeable, and jing can be round and alive. If breath is held or sealed, qi will be stagnant and accumulate.

息調得宜，氣則順轉，勁能圓活。息如閉塞，氣則滯積，勁必呆死。

At the beginning of training, yi is on the breathing, qi will then follow. Later, yi is not on the breathing (qi) but on the opponent. Yi is forming, qi will grow, jing will be emitted naturally, and reach to the point where when yi arrives jing arrives also.

初行之，意在息，氣隨之。爾後，意不在氣，而在彼。意孕而氣生，勁自然而發。而終於意到勁亦到之功效。

The qi of the heng-ha sounds is determined by breathing. When breathing is right, then the Spirit of Vitality rises, and qi will be full, and emitting and withdrawing jings can reach their highest.

哼哈之氣制於息。息正則精神振，氣可沛然。收發之勁亦可達峰。

5-6. Taijiquan Poetry and Songs

Sun Zi's Fighting Strategies 孫子戰略
Sun Wu (557 BCE) 孫武

Sun Wu, also known as Sun Zi (Mister Sun, 孫子, and in the West as Sun Tzu), was a very famous strategist who lived around 557 BCE. His book *Sun Zi's Fighting Strategies* (*Sun Zi Bing Fa*, 孫子兵法, often translated as *The Art of War*) has been studied by Chinese soldiers for centuries and has become required reading in most military schools throughout the world. Although phrased in terms of battles and troop movements, the book applies equally well to individual conflicts.

Knowing the opponent and knowing yourself, a hundred battles without a loss. Not knowing the opponent but knowing yourself, one victory one loss. Not knowing the opponent and not knowing yourself, every battle will be lost.

知彼知己，百戰不殆。不知彼而知己，一勝一負。不知彼，不知己，每戰每敗。

In a battle, if you know your opponent and yourself, you will be able to set up your strategy according to the situation and win every time. When you know yourself but do not know the enemy, you are at the mercy of chance and have only a fifty-fifty chance of winning. If you know neither yourself nor your opponent, then you will lose for sure.

Whenever in a battle, use regularity to combine [engage], [but use] surprise to win. Therefore, the one who is good in using surprise, [his strategy] is limitless like the heaven and earth, [his wisdom] is not dry, [it is] like a river or stream. The conduct of battle is nothing else but using regularity and surprise. The exchange of surprise and regularity [is] limitless. Surprise and regularity mutually grow, like a cycle with no end. Who can limit it [figure it out]?

凡戰者，　以正合，　以奇勝。故善出奇者，　無窮如天地，　不竭如江河。戰勢不過奇正，　奇正之變，　不可勝窮也。奇正相生，　如循環之無端，　孰能窮之？

Regularity, in the sense of both fixed organization and standard operating procedures (SOPs), is yang. Surprise, or change, is yin. Regularity in organization and SOPs allows your units to combine and work together for greater strength. Regularity also means developing routines and techniques that allow you to effectively develop and use maximum power. However, if you always follow these routines, your opponent can develop ways to defeat them, so you must also use surprise, or changes in the routines, to keep the enemy off balance so he cannot effectively mobilize his strength. In individual training and fighting, you must develop set routines, but you must never be bound by them. You may do something several times so that the opponent expects you to do it again, but then you must change in order to surprise him and win. If you can skillfully exchange regularity and surprise (which can be called substantial and insubstantial), you will be able to respond to the opponent's actions with a limitless variety of actions.

Therefore, when using soldiers the ultimate shape is to have no shape. If there is no shape, then it is like a deep mountain torrent which cannot be fathomed, and [even] a wise person cannot set up a strategy [against you]. Everyone [thinks he] understands how I win the victories from the shape [they can see], but they don't know the shape of how I really win the victory. Therefore [I] do not repeat [my] victories, and [my] response to shapes [situations] is unlimited.

故形兵之極。　至於無形。無形則深潤不能窺，　智者不能謀 。人皆知我所以勝之形，而莫知吾所以制勝之形。故其戰勝不復，　而應形於無窮。

When fighting, the ultimate strategy is to seem to have no strategy. If the opponent cannot determine what your strategy is, or if it seems that you have no strategy, then he will not be able to devise a strategy against you. If the enemy thinks he knows me well, he will be able to set up a good strategy and will seem to be winning. However, because my strategy is actually shapeless, he has been basing his actions on illusion, and he will lose in the end. When I attack, he thinks he knows what I plan (my shape), and he can counterattack. However, it is only a feint used to draw him out and make him act. Once his plans have taken shape, I base my strategy on that shape and act accordingly. Because my strategy is not tied to any particular form, it can change through an endless number of variations and never repeat itself.

In conclusion, soldiers [strategies] are like water. The shape [nature] of water [is to] avoid the high and flow to the low. The shape [correct disposition] of soldiers [is to] avoid the substantial and attack the insubstantial. Water comes over into a stream due to the shape of the ground, soldiers gain the victory through corresponding to the enemy['s shape]. Therefore, soldiers do not have a fixed status [posture, disposition] and water does not have a fixed shape. [Being] able to change corresponding to the enemy's strategy and win the battle is called Shen [Spiritual Enlightenment].

夫兵像水。水之形, 避高而趨下。兵之形, 避實而擊虛。水因地而制流, 兵因敵而制勝。故兵無常勢, 水無常形。能因敵變化而取勝者, 謂之神。

Water avoids the high and flows to the low. When conducting soldiers or fighting, you must avoid the substantial (strong points) and attack the insubstantial (weak points). Just as water can become a powerful stream by following the shape of the land, so too can soldiers become a strong attacking force by responding to and corresponding to the shape of the enemy. Basing your strategy on the strategy of the opponent is the way to victory and is considered Spiritual Enlightenment. In taijiquan this is called giving up yourself and following the opponent. If I do not resist the opponent and stick to him wherever he moves, he will never be able to find me and effectively attack me, but I will always know where he is and what he is planning. Because of this, I can defeat him with certainty.

Strategies

1. The Strategy of Movement and Stillness 動靜略
Author Unknown

The ultimate of movement is stillness, the ultimate of stillness is movement. To move is to generate stillness, and to be still is to generate movement. Therefore, [if you] use stillness as movement, [your] movement will be stronger every day. [If you] use movement as movement, [your] movement will weaken daily. [If you] use movement to drive stillness, [it is] calm and long. [If you] use stillness to drive the movement, [it is] vigorous and strong.

動極則靜, 靜極則動。動以成靜, 故以靜為動, 其動日強。以動為動, 其動日弱, 而以動馭靜, 靜而可久。以靜馭動, 動而可大。

The ultimate of movement happens when your heart (mind) is still. The mind can then see clearly, and your actions can be accurately apportioned to the opponent's actions. The ultimate of stillness is when you can act correctly while maintaining a quiet mind. Taijiquan is considered meditation in motion, and as you practice, you gradually become more and more centered and peaceful. After a while, your mind can be absolutely still while your body moves seemingly by itself in response to your opponent's actions. The more you practice centering and quieting the mind, the stronger your movements will become, because you can see clearly and act efficiently. If, on the other hand, you practice the movements as movements, they will seem to become weaker, because you have trained yourself to do the movements independent of what the opponent is actually doing. Your movements will be forced and stiff, rather than natural and smooth. If you use your physical training as a way to train your mind, your mind will become calm, and your attention span will grow. If you remain calm and centered, your movements will be strong because you can concentrate all of your force, and you will be able to vary and adapt them to the circumstances.

2. The Strategy of Advance and Withdraw 進退略
Author Unknown

> *[If you] use an advance as an advance, the advance will not be defensible. [If you] use a withdrawal as a withdrawal, the withdrawal will be defeated. [If you] use a withdrawal as an advance, the withdrawal will create an advance. [If you] use an advance as a withdrawal, advance two, withdraw one. Advance and withdrawal must be mutually balanced. Especially important is the [waiting for the right] opportunity. When the opportunity is missed, then advance and withdrawal are both difficult.*

以進為進，其進不守。以退為退，其退必敗。以退為進，退以成進。以進為退，進以成退。進之者二，退之者一。進退相衡，尤貴機先。機先一失，則進退兩難矣。

This paragraph emphasizes the importance of deception. You must keep the opponent confused so that he never knows if what you seem to be doing is what you actually are doing. If he can see clearly that you are advancing, he may be able to react effectively and defeat you. If he can see clearly that you are retreating, he can press his attack and defeat you. If you want to advance, pretend to withdraw, and your advance will take him by surprise. Likewise, if you want to withdraw, you must first advance to that you will be able to safely withdraw. To win a battle, it is usually more important to advance than to withdraw, but the two must be balanced in the right proportion. In all of this, it is most important to act only at the correct time. You must wait for the right opportunity and then act, for if you miss the opportunity, it may not come again, and you will surely lose. The taijiquan classics refer to this as grasping the moment and seizing the opportunity.

3. The Strategy of Long and Short 長短略
Author Unknown

To use the long to attack the short is to battle with advantage. To use the short to attack the long is a battle [that needs] wisdom. Use the enemy's long to attack the enemy's short and use the enemy's short to attack the enemy's long, then it is called enlightened combat.

以長攻短，是為鬥力。以短攻長，是為鬥智。以敵之長，攻敵之短。以敵之短，攻敵之長。則為鬥之以神。

Here "long" means advantage, and "short" means disadvantage. For example, if you are strong and use your strength to defeat a weaker person, your strength is called long. Therefore, if you have an advantage, you will naturally use this advantage to defeat the enemy. However, if you are the disadvantaged side, you will not be able to defeat your enemy through your weakness, so you must use your wisdom in a fight. To use your opponent's advantage to defeat his weakness and to use his weakness to attack his advantage, this is called fighting with enlightenment. For example, if your enemy is strong and muscular, he may be slow, so you must use your speed to defeat his strength. Or if your enemy has a long weapon, he will not be effective in short-range defense, so you should specialize in short-range attack. You can use his long against his short if, for example, he specializes in long-range kicking. If you stay at long range, you will encourage him to confidently attack. This will give you the opportunity to slip past his attack and attack at short range. If you are able to do all this, it is called enlightened combat.

4. The Strategy of Hard and Soft 剛柔略
Dr. Yang, Jwing-Ming 楊俊敏

When using the soft to subdue the hard, the soft must be skillful and adaptable. Using soft to control soft is harder than hard. Using hard against hard, skill and li [both] stagnant and sluggish. If you use hard to defeat soft, your power and skill will be dull and hard to apply. Hard and soft mutually assisting and cooperating is the best strategy.

以柔克剛，柔必巧熟。以柔制柔，難上加難。以剛應剛，技力遲鈍。以剛克柔，技死難展。剛柔相濟，乃為上策。

If you use the soft against the hard, you must be skillful in yielding, adhering, and sticking. Like a snake wrapping and coiling around a branch, you must adapt to whatever the opponent does. When you meet an opponent who is also skilled at softness, then it will be extremely hard to defeat him. Your skill must be better and higher than his, otherwise you will not be able to apply your techniques. If you use hard to resist a hard attack, your actions will be stagnant and your power sluggish. If you try to use hard to subdue the soft, your techniques will be dead and impossible to apply. The best approach is to exchange hard and soft properly. This mutual assistance and cooperation will make your techniques alive and useful.

5. The Strategy of Fast and Slow 快慢略

Dr. Yang, Jwing-Ming 楊俊敏

When using the slow to defeat the fast, qi must be emphasized. When using fast to beat the slow, the yi goes first. When fast and slow are used at the right time, and yi and qi exchange skillfully, it is called light and agile (qing-ling).

以慢敵快，以氣為重。以快侮慢，以意為先。快慢應得時，意氣轉得巧，是為輕靈。

When you use the slow to defeat the fast, you must be calm, and your qi must be full. Only when your qi is full and stimulated are you able to generate the power needed to bounce away attacks. Then it is like a beach ball bouncing away a fast punch. However, when you intend to use speed to beat the slow, your yi must always go first. That means that while you are defending, your yi is already on attacking; and while you are attacking, your yi is already aware of the opponent's attack. However, the best fighting strategy is to match his speed so that fast follows the fast and slow follows the slow. If you can do this while skillfully exchanging your emphasis on yi and qi, your movements and thinking will be light and agile.

Chapter 6: Conclusion

This book can give the reader only general concepts and guidelines of taijiquan bare-hand training. All the training methods are only examples. There are many other training methods that can be used to develop the taijiquan techniques to a higher level. These training methods should be researched, studied, and experimented with by the practitioner. In the course of the training, you should repeatedly go back to *Tai Chi Chuan Martial Power*, 3rd edition, especially the poetry and songs in the appendix. This way you will be able to combine both theory and practical techniques.

In China, there is a proverb: "There is a sky above a sky, and a talent above a talent" (人外有人，天外有天). This means that you should never be satisfied with your ability. There is always someone out there who is higher than you and can be your teacher. You should continue your search for a higher talent and at the same time practice ceaselessly. One day you will find you are a great master with a humble mind and abundant taijiquan knowledge.

Generally, there are a few rules that can help you find a qualified taijiquan master. Before you make up your mind, you should first ask the following:

- Does he know general taijiquan history? What is his background?
- Does this taijiquan master understand the taijiquan principles and explain them well?
- Does he know yi, qi, and jing well?
- Does he know the applications of every form?
- Does he have a good training schedule?
- How often does he communicate with his students?

Once you are satisfied about these things, you should then request a free trial lesson. This will allow you to directly feel the mood and the learning environment, and you will be able to make a sensible decision.

Acknowledgments

Acknowledgments (1986)

Thanks to Eng-Lok Lim for the photography, Eric Hoffman for proofing the manuscript and for contributing many valuable suggestions and discussions, and John Casagrande Jr. for his drawings. Special thanks to Alan Dougall for his editing, and a very special thanks to the artist Nian-Fu Zong for his beautiful calligraphy on the front pages of both volumes.

Second Edition (1996)

In this new edition, I would like to express many thanks to Tim Comrie, Kathy K. Yang, and Nicholas C. Yang for general help; to Kain M. Sanderson and Jeff Grace for proofing; and to Andrew Murray for his editing. Thanks also to Deborah Clark for her new cover design.

Third Edition (2016)

The publisher wishes to thank Axie Breen for cover design, Leslie Takao for copyediting, T. G. LaFredo for editorial management, and Tim Comrie for project management.

Appendix A

Yang-Style Taijiquan 37 Postures

1. Grasp Sparrow's Tail, Right and Left (Lan Que Wei, 攬雀尾)
2. Wardoff (Peng, 掤)
3. Rollback (Lu, 挴)
4. Press (Ji, 擠)
5. Push (An, 按)
6. Single Whip (Dan Bian, 單鞭)
7. Lift Hands and Lean Forward (Ti Shou Shang Shi, 提手上勢)
8. The Crane Spreads Its Wings (Bai He Liang Chi, 白鶴亮翅)
9. Brush Knee and Step Forward (Lou Xi Yao Bu, 摟膝拗步)
10. Play the Guitar (Shou Hui Pi Pa, 手揮琵琶)
11. Twist Body and Circle Fist (Pie Shen Chui, 撇身捶)
12. Step Forward, Deflect Downward, Parry, and Punch (Jin Bu Ban Lan Chui, 進步搬攔捶)
13. Seal Tightly (Ru Feng Si Bi, 如封似閉)
14. Embrace Tiger and Return to the Mountain (Bao Hu Gui Shan, 抱虎歸山) Transition Form between the Parts (Guo Du Shi, 過渡勢)
15. Punch under the Elbow (Zhou Di Kan Chui, 肘底看捶)
16. Step Back and Repulse Monkey (Dao Nian Hou, 倒撵猴)
17. Diagonal Flying (Xie Fei Shi, 斜飛勢)
18. Pick Up Needle from Sea Bottom (Hai Di Lao Zhen, 海底撈針)
19. Fan Back (Shan Tong Bei, 扇通背)
20. Wave Hands in the Clouds (Yun Shou, 雲手)
21. Stand High to Search Out the Horse (Gao Tan Ma, 高探馬)
22. Separate Foot (Fen Jiao, 分腳)
23. Kick with Heel (Deng Jiao, 蹬腳)
24. Step Forward and Strike Down with the Fist (Jin Bu Zai Chui, 進步栽捶)
25. Strike the Tiger (Da Hu, 打虎)
26. Attack the Ears with the Fists (Shuang Feng Guan Er, 雙風貫耳)

27. Wild Horses Shear the Mane (Ye Ma Fen Zong, 野馬分鬃)
28. Fair Lady Weaves with Shuttle (Yu Nu Chuan Suo, 玉女穿梭)
29. Lower the Snake Body (She Shen Xia Shi, 蛇身下勢)
30. Golden Rooster Stands on One Leg (Jin Ji Du Li, 金雞獨立)
31. White Snake Turns Body and Spits Poison (Bai She Tu Xin, 白蛇吐信)
32. Cross Hands (Shi Zi Shou, 十字手)
33. Brush Knee and Punch Down (Lou Xi Zhi Dang Chui, 摟膝指襠捶)
34. Step Forward to Seven Stars (Shang Bu Qi Xing, 上步七星)
35. Step Back to Ride the Tiger (Tui Bu Kua Hu, 退步跨虎)
36. Turn Body and Sweep Lotus (Zhuan Shen Bai Lian, 轉身擺蓮)
37. Draw the Bow and Shoot the Tiger (Wan Gong She Hu, 彎守射虎)

Appendix B

Yang-Style Taijiquan Fighting Set

1. Step Forward for Punch (Shang Bu Chui, 上步捶)
2. Raise Hands to the Up Posture (Ti Shou Shang Shi, 提手上勢)
3. Step Forward, Intercept, and Punch (Shang Bu Lan Chui, 上步攔捶)
4. Deflect and Punch (Ban Chui, 搬捶)
5. Step Forward and Left Shoulder Stroke (Shang Bu Zuo Kao, 上步左靠)
6. Strike the Tiger (Right) (You Da Hu, 右打虎)
7. Left Elbow Strike (Zuo Zhou Da, 左肘打)
8. Push to the Left and Right Elbow Stroke (Zuo Tui You Kao, 左推右靠)
9. Withdraw the Step and Strike the Tiger (Left) (Che Bu You Da Hu, 撤步右打虎)
10. Right Downward Strike (You Xia Chui, 右下捶)
11. Raise Hands to the Up Posture (Ti Shou Shang Shi, 提手上勢)
12. Turn the Body and Push (Zhuan Shen An, 轉身按)
13. Right Swinging-Body Strike (You Pie Shen Chui, 右撇身捶)
14. Intercept and Punch, One (Ban Chui Yi Shi, 搬捶一勢)
15. Intercept and Punch, Two (Ban Chui Er Shi, 搬捶二勢)
16. Wild Horses Shear the Mane (Left) (Zuo Ye Ma Fen Zong, 左野馬分鬃)
17. Strike the Tiger (Right) (You Da Hu, 右打虎)
18. Turn the Body, Withdraw the Step, and Execute Rollback (Zhuan Shen Che Bu Lu, 轉身撤步擺)
19. Step Forward and Press (Left) (Shang Bu Zuo Ji, 上步左擠)
20. Turn the Body and Press (Left) (Zhuan Shen Zuo Ji, 轉身左擠)
21. Double Dividing and Heel Kick (Shuang Fen Deng Jiao, 雙分蹬腳)
22. Punch the Groin (Zhi Dang Chui, 指襠捶)
23. Step Forward to Pluck and Rend (Shang Bu Cai Lie, 上步採挒)
24. Fair Lady Weaves with Shuttle, One (Yu Nu Chuan Suo Yi Shi, 玉女穿梭一勢)
25. Fair Lady Weaves with Shuttle, Two (Yu Nu Chuan Suo Er Shi, 玉女穿梭二勢)
26. White Crane Spreads Its Wings (Bai He Liang Chi, 白鶴亮翅)
27. Left Shoulder Stroke (Zuo Kao, 左靠)

28. Execute Rollback against the Shoulder (Lu Bi, 捋臂)

29. Turn the Body to Rend the Shoulder (Zhuan Shen Lie Bi, 轉身挒臂)

30. Turn the Body to Execute Rollback (Zhuan Shen Lu, 轉身捋)

31. Two Winds Pass through the Ears (Shuang Feng Guan Er, 雙風貫耳)

32. Double Push (Shuang An, 雙按)

33. Single Whip (Dan Bian, 單鞭)

34. Right Push (You Tui, 右推)

35. File the Shoulder (Right) (You Cuo Bi, 右挫臂)

36. Follow the Posture and Push (Shun Shi An, 順勢按)

37. Neutralize and Strike with Right Palm (Hua Da You Zhang, 化打右掌)

38. Neutralize and Push (Hua Tui, 化推)

39. Neutralize and Strike with Right Elbow (Hua Da You Zhou, 化打右肘)

40. Pluck and Rend (Cai Lie, 採挒)

41. Exchange Steps and Execute Rollback (Huan Bu Lu, 換步捋)

42. Step Forward and Press (Shang Bu Ji, 上步擠)

43. Exchange Steps and Execute Rollback (Huan Bu Lu, 換步捋)

44. Strike the Tiger (Right) (You Da Hu, 右打虎)

45. Turn the Body, Step Backward, and Execute Rollback (Zhuan Shen Che Bu Lu, 轉身撤步捋)

46. Step Forward and Press to the Left (Shang Bu Zuo Ji, 上步左擠)

47. Return with Press (Hui Ji, 回擠)

48. Exchange Steps and Shoulder Stroke (Right) (Huan Bu You Kao, 換步右靠)

49. Turn the Body to Fly Diagonally (Zhuan Shen Xie Fei Shi, 轉身斜飛勢)

50. Right Elbow Strike (You Zhou Da, 右肘打)

51. Turn the Body for Rooster Standing on One Leg (Zhuan Shen Jin Ji Du Li, 轉身金雞獨立)

52. Downward Neutralization (Xia Hua, 下化)

53. Heel Kick (Deng Jiao, 蹬腳)

54. Turn the Body, Step Forward, and Strike (Zhuan Shen Shang Bu Kao, 轉身上步靠)

55. Execute Rollback against Left Arm (Lu Zuo Bi, 捋左臂

56. Turn the Body and Right Kick (Zhuan Shen You Fen Jiao, 轉身右分腳)

57. Double Dividing and Embrace the Knee (Right) (Shuang Fen You Lou Xi, 雙分右摟膝)

58. Turn the Body and Left Kick (Zhuan Shen Zuo Fen Jiao, 轉身左分腳)

59. Double Dividing and Embrace the Knee (Left) (Shuang Fen Zuo Lou Xi, 雙分左摟膝)

60. Change Hands and Right Shoulder Stroke (Huan Shou You Kao, 換手右靠)

61. Return Right Elbow Stroke (Hui You Kao, 回右靠)

62. Step Forward and Grasp the Sparrow's Tail (Left) (Shang Bu Zuo Lan Que Wei, 上步左攬雀尾)

63. Wave Hands in Clouds (Right) (You Yun Shou, 右雲手)

64. Step Forward and Grasp the Sparrow's Tail (Right) (Shang Bu You Lan Que Wei, 上步右攬雀尾)

65. Wave Hands in Clouds (Left) (Zuo Yun Shou, 左雲手)

66. Divide Upward, Press, and Downward Heel Kick (Shang Fen Ji Xia Deng Tui, 上分擠下蹬腿)

67. Low Hook Kick (Xia Gou Tui, 下勾腿)

68. Turn the Body to Sweep Lotus (Zhuan Shen Bai Lian, 轉身擺蓮)

69. Left Elbow Stroke (Zuo Kao, 左靠)

70. Hook Hand and Snake Creeps Down (Diao Shou She Shen Xia Shi, 刁手蛇身下勢)

71. Diagonal Flying (Right) (You Xie Fei Shi, 右斜飛勢)

72. Strike the Tiger (Left) (Zuo Da Hu, 左打虎)

73. Double Dividing and Push Down (Shuang Fen Xia An, 雙分下按)

74. Step Back and Repulse Monkey (Dao Nian Hou, 倒攆猴)

75. Left Push (Zuo An, 左按)

76. Step Back and Repulse Monkey (Dao Nian Hou, 倒攆猴)

77. Right Push (You An, 右按)

78. Repulse Monkey (Dao Nian Hou, 倒攆猴)

79. Right Palm Strike (You Zhang Pai, 右掌拍)

80. Step Forward to Seven Stars (Shang Bu Qi Xing, 上步七星)

81. Pick Up Needle from Sea Bottom (Hai Di Zhen, 海底針)

82. Fan Back (Shan Tong Bei, 扇通背)

83. Pluck Right (You Cai, 右採)

84. Draw the Bow and Shoot the Tiger (Wan Gong She Hu, 彎弓射虎)

85. Neutralize Up and Press Forward (Xia Hua Ping Ji, 下化平擠)

86. Punch under the Elbow (Zhou Di Kan Chui, 肘底看捶)

87. Cross Hands (Shi Zi Shou, 十字手)

88. Embrace Tiger and Return to the Mountain (Bao Hu Gui Shan, 抱虎歸山)

Appendix C

Translation and Glossary of Chinese Terms

an (按). Push. A technique for pushing or striking the opponent. It is one of the four directions of the eight basic taijiquan fighting techniques, which correspond to the eight trigrams (bagua, 八卦).

bagua (八卦). The eight trigrams. The *Yi Jing*, a book of philosophy, lists eight basic principles that are derived from yin and yang, and in turn give rise to other variations. These eight principles are each represented by three broken and/or straight lines known as trigrams (see *Yi Jing*). In taijiquan the trigrams correspond to the basic techniques peng, lu, ji, an, cai, lie, zhou, and kao.

baguazhang (八卦掌). Eight trigrams palm. One of the internal Chinese martial styles, based on the bagua theory. It emphasizes the application of palm techniques and circular movements. Baguazhang was created by Dong, Hai-Chuan (董海川) in the nineteenth century.

Bai He (白鶴). White Crane. A style of southern Shaolin gongfu that imitates the fighting techniques of the crane.

cai (採). Pluck. A technique for unbalancing the opponent or pulling him into an exposed position. One of the four corners of the eight basic taijiquan fighting techniques.

chang chuan (changquan) (長拳). Long fist or long sequence. When it means long fist, it is a northern Shaolin Chinese martial style that specializes in kicking techniques. When it means long sequence, it refers to taijiquan and implies that the taijiquan sequence is long and flowing like a river.

Chang, San-Feng (Zhang, San-Feng) (張三豐). Said to be the creator of taijiquan in the Song dynasty (960–1279 CE) (宋朝). However, there is no certain documentary proof of this.

Cheng, Gin-Gsao (曾金灶). Dr. Yang, Jwing-Ming's White Crane master.

chin na (qin na) (擒拿). Grasp and control. An aspect of Chinese martial arts training, chin na specializes in controlling the enemy through "misplacing the joint" (cuo gu, 錯骨), "dividing the muscle" (fen jin, 分筋), "sealing the breath" (bi qi, 閉氣), and "cavity press" (dian xue, 點穴).

chuan (quan) (拳). Fist. This term in Chinese martial arts is also used to denote a gongfu style (e.g., Shaolin quan or taijiquan) or a sequence (e.g., lian bu quan [連步拳] or gong li quan [功力拳]).

chuang (窗). Window. The open space of an opponent that can be used for attacking.

da lu (大攦). Large rollback. Rollback is one of the eight basic taijiquan fighting techniques and is a method of leading the opponent's attack past you. There are two versions—large and small rollback. Da lu also refers to a two-person pushing-hands exercise that concentrates on using the four "corners" (cai, lie, zhou, kao), as well as the four "directions" (peng, lu, ji, an).

da shou (搭手). Folding hands. Two opponents exchanging hand techniques. It is called pushing hands in taijiquan or bridge hands (qiao shou, 橋手) in other styles.

dan tian (丹田). Field of elixir. There are three dan tian in the body: the brain, the solar plexus area, and the lower abdomen. Taijiquan is primarily interested in the lower dan tian. It is considered the reservoir of qi and is located approximately one and one-half inches below the navel and about a third of the way toward the spine. In acupuncture, this point is known as qihai (氣海) (sea of qi).

di chuang (地窗). Ground window. The opening of a lower section of an opponent's body that offers you an opportunity for attack.

ding bu tui shou (定步推手). Stationary pushing hands. Taijiquan hand technique drills in which both partners are stationary.

dong bu tui shou (動步推手). Moving pushing hands. Taijiquan hand technique drills in which both partners are moving and stepping.

dui shou (對手). Opposing hands. Hand drills practiced by two or more persons. Also called bridge hands (qiao shou, 橋手) or folding hands (da shou, 搭手).

Emei (峨嵋). Name of a mountain in Sichuan Province (四川省), China.

Eng-Lok Lim (林應祿). A friend and student of Dr. Yang, Jwing-Ming.

gongfu (kung fu) (功夫). Energy-time. Anything that takes time and energy to master is called gongfu. In recent times it has come to mean Chinese martial arts.

guoshu (kuoshu) (國術). National technique. The name for Chinese martial arts used by Chiang, Kai-Shek (蔣介石) since 1927, and still used in Taiwan. Mainland China uses the term *wushu* (武術).

ha (哈). One of the two sounds used in taijiquan and other Chinese martial styles. The ha sound is positive (yang) and is used to raise the spirit of vitality (jing shen, 精神), enabling power to reach its maximum.

hai di (海底). Sea bottom. The groin area. The head is called heavenly cover (tian ling gai, 天靈蓋).

heng (哼). One of the two sounds used in taijiquan. When done on inhalation, the heng sound is purely negative (yin). It condenses the yi and qi into the bone marrow. When done on exhalation, heng is negative with some positive. This allows you to attack while conserving some energy.

jin bu (進步). Step forward. One of the five basic strategic movements of taijiquan.

jing (經). The main qi (energy) channels. In the human body there are twelve pairs of these channels, which are related to the internal organs.

jing (精). Essence. What is left after something has been refined and purified. In Chinese medicine, jing can mean semen, but it generally refers to the basic substance of the body that the qi and spirit enliven.

Jing Shen (精神). Essence of the spirit; spirit of vitality. A person with a strong Jing Shen is active, vigorous, and concentrated.

jiuwei (Co-15) (鳩尾). An acupuncture cavity belonging to the conception vessel.

kao (靠). Bump. A technique using the shoulder, hip, thigh, back, or any other part of the body to bump the opponent off balance. One of the four corners of the eight basic taijiquan fighting techniques.

Kao, Tao (高濤). Dr. Yang, Jwing-Ming's first taijiquan master.

kong men (空門). Empty door. The opening space you step into to attack an opponent.

kou jue (口訣). Mouth secret words. Secrets that have been passed down orally.

kung fu (gongfu) (功夫). Energy-time. Anything that takes time and energy to master is called gongfu. In recent times it has come to mean Chinese martial arts.

kuoshu (guoshu) (國術). National technique. The name for Chinese martial arts used by Chiang, Kai-Shek (蔣介石) since 1927, and still used in Taiwan. Mainland China uses the term *wushu* (武術).

leng jing (冷勁). Cold jing. A sudden jing manifestation (i.e., an attack) that surprises your opponent.

li (力). Muscular power; strength.

Li, Mao-Ching (李茂清). Dr. Yang, Jwing-Ming's Long Fist master.

Liang dynasty (梁代). A dynasty in Chinese history (502–557 CE).

lie (e). Split or rend. The use of two opposing forces to lock or unbalance the opponent. One of the four corners of the eight basic taijiquan fighting techniques.

lu (擺). Rollback. A technique for leading the opponent's attack past you. One of the four directions of the eight basic taijiquan fighting techniques.

lu dao (擺倒). Use rollback to make someone fall.

luo (絡). Branches. The numerous tiny qi channels that extend from the major channels (jing, 經) and allow the qi to reach from the skin to the marrow.

mo (摸). Smear. A technique from double pushing-hands training.

na (拿). To control or to grab. A pushing hand technique that specializes in controlling the opponent's joints.

neiguan (P-6) (內關). An acupuncture cavity belonging to the pericardium channel (心包絡經).

Nian-Fu Zong (蹤念富). A scholar and calligrapher in China who wrote the calligraphy on the cover of this book.

pan xi (盤吸). Coil suction. A taijiquan jing that specializes in sticking-adhering to part of an opponent's body.

peng (掤). Wardoff. A technique for bouncing the opponent's force back in the direction it came. One of the four directions of the eight basic taijiquan fighting techniques.

qi (chi) (氣). The "intrinsic energy" that circulates in all living things.

qi xing zhen (七星陣). Seven star tactics. Refers to ways of positioning and moving troops in battle.

qiao shou (橋手). Bridge hands. It is called pushing hands in taijiquan or folding hands (da shou, 搭手) in other styles.

qigong (chi kung) (氣功). A type of gongfu training that specializes in building up the qi circulation in the body for health and/or martial purposes.

qin na (chin na) (擒拿). Grasp and control. An aspect of Chinese martial arts training, chin na specializes in controlling the enemy through "misplacing the joint" (cuo gu, 錯骨), "dividing the muscle" (fen jin, 分筋), "sealing the breath" (bi qi, 閉氣), and "cavity press" (dian xue, 點穴).

qing ling (輕靈). Lightness and agility. These words are often used to describe the motion of monkeys—responsive, controlled, and able to move quickly.

quchi (LI-11) (曲池). An acupuncture cavity belonging to the large intestine channel (大腸經).

ruan bian (軟鞭). Soft whip. Usually made from leather.

ruan ying bian (軟硬鞭). Soft-hard whip. Usually made from rattan.

rugen (S-18) (乳根). An acupuncture cavity belonging to the stomach channel (胃經).

ruzhong (S-17) (乳中). An acupuncture cavity belonging to the stomach channel (胃經).

san shi qi shi (三十七勢). Thirty-seven postures. According to historical records, one of the predecessors of taijiquan.

Shaolin (少林). The name of a Buddhist temple, built in 377 CE, which later became a Chinese martial arts training center.

shen (神). Spirit. The consciousness within which the mind and thought function.

Song dynasty (宋代). A dynasty in Chinese history (960–1278 CE).

Sun Zi (孫子). Mister Sun. Sun Wu (孫武). A famous strategist who lived around 557 BCE. He wrote the book *Sun Zi's Fighting Strategies* (*Sun Zi Bing Fa*, 孫子兵法). This book is commonly translated as *The Art of War*.

taiji (太極). Grand ultimate. The state in which opposites (known as yin and yang) are generated.

taijiquan (太極拳). Grand ultimate fist. A Chinese internal martial style.

Taipei (臺北). The capital of Taiwan.

Taiwan (臺灣). An island located southeast of China; often called Formosa.

Tamkang College (淡江學院). The college from which Dr. Yang, Jwing-Ming obtained his BS in physics. This college is now called Tamkang University.

tian chuang (天窗). Sky window. The opening of the upper section of an opponent's body that offers you the opportunity to attack.

tian ling gai (天靈蓋). Heaven spirit cover. It means the top of the head.

tianshu (S-25) (天樞). An acupuncture cavity belonging to the stomach channel (胃經).

tong bei yuan (tong bi yuan) (通背猿) (通臂猿). Reach-the-back apes or reachable-arm apes. Apes with long arms.

tui bu (退步). Step backward. One of the five basic strategic movements of taijiquan.

tuo tian (托天). Supporting the heavens. A form of qigong training used to increase the strength and endurance of the legs and also build up qi in the spine.

tui shou (推手). Pushing hands. A taijiquan hand technique drill.

Wu Song (武松). A fictional hero of the Song dynasty (960–1278 CE) (宋朝).

Wudang (武當). A mountain located to the south of Shi Yan town, in Hubei Province (十堰市, 湖北省), China. It is believed that a number of Daoist martial arts, such as taijiquan and Wudang, were created in this area.

wushu (武術). Martial technique. Chinese martial arts were once called wu yi (武藝) (martial arts), and the techniques of wu yi were called wushu (martial techniques). In 1927, the name was changed to guoshu (國術) (kuoshu) but was changed back to wushu in 1949. It is still called guoshu (kuoshu) in Taiwan.

xiao lu (小捋). Small rollback. A taijiquan pushing-hands technique.

xiaohai (SI-8) (小海). An acupuncture cavity belonging to the small intestine channel.

xin (心). Heart. In Chinese, it often means "mind." It refers to an intention, idea, or thought that has not been expressed.

yang (陽). The positive pole of taiji (grand ultimate), the other pole being yin (negative). The Chinese believe that everything follows from the interaction of yin and yang.

Yang, Jwing-Ming (楊俊敏). Author of this book.

yao duan (拗斷). To break.

yao zhe (拗折). To break.

yi (意). Mind. It is commonly expressed as xin-yi. Xin (心) is an idea and yi (意) is the expression of this idea. Therefore, yi by itself can be translated as "mind."

yin (陰). The negative pole of taiji (grand ultimate). See also yang.

ying bian (硬鞭). Hard whip. A type of short weapon in ancient China.

yingchuang (S-16) (膺窗). An acupuncture cavity belonging to the stomach channel (胃經).

yongquan (K-1) (湧泉). An acupuncture cavity belonging to the kidney channel (腎經).

you kong men (右空門). Right empty door. The opening on your opponent's right through which you can enter for an attack.

you pan (右盼). Right look (look to the right). It implies beware of your right-hand side.

Zhang, San-Feng (Chang, San-Feng) (張三豐). Said to be the creator of taijiquan in the Song dynasty (宋朝) (960–1279 CE). However, there is no certain documentary proof of this.

zhong ding (中定). Central equilibrium. One of the five basic strategic movements.

zhou (肘). Elbow. The technique of striking or neutralizing with the elbow. One of the four corners of the eight basic taijiquan fighting techniques.

zou bagua (走八卦). Walking bagua. Chinese martial arts training in which a practitioner walks in a circle.

zuo gu (左顧). Beware of the left. One of the five fundamental strategic movements that correspond to the five elements.

zuo kong men (左空門). Left empty door. The opening on your opponent's left through which you can enter for an attack.

Index

About the Author

Yang, Jwing-Ming, PhD 楊俊敏博士

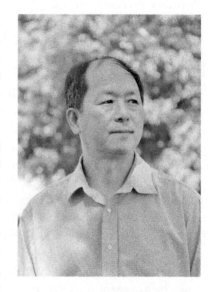

Dr. Yang, Jwing-Ming was born on August 11, 1946, in Xinzhu Xian (新竹縣), Taiwan (台灣), Republic of China (中華民國). He started his wushu (武術) (gongfu or kung fu, 功夫) training at the age of fifteen under the Shaolin White Crane (Bai He, 少林白鶴) master Cheng, Gin-Gsao (曾金社灶). Master Cheng originally learned Taizuquan (太祖拳) as a child from his grandfather. When Master Cheng was fifteen years old, he started learning White Crane from Master Jin, Shao-Feng (金紹峰), and followed him for twenty-three years until Master Jin's death.

In thirteen years of study (1961–1974) under Master Cheng, Dr. Yang became an expert in the White Crane style of Chinese martial arts, which includes both the use of bare hands and of various weapons such as saber, staff, spear, trident, two short rods, and many others. With the same master, he also studied White Crane qigong (氣功), chin na (or qin na, 擒拿), tui na (推拿) and dian xue massages (點穴按摩), and herbal treatment.

At the age of sixteen Dr. Yang began the study of Yang-style taijiquan (楊氏太極拳) under Master Kao Tao (高濤). After learning from Master Kao, Dr. Yang continued his study and research of taijiquan with several masters and senior practitioners such as Master Li, Mao-Ching (李茂清) and Mr. Wilson Chen (陳威仲伸) in Taipei (台北). Master Li learned his taijiquan from the well-known Master Han, Ching-Tang (韓慶堂), and Mr. Chen learned his taijiquan from Master Chang, Xiang-San (張祥三). Dr. Yang has mastered the taijiquan bare-hand sequence, pushing hands, the two-man fighting sequence, taiji sword, taiji saber, and taiji qigong.

When Dr. Yang was eighteen years old, he entered Tamkang College (淡江學院) in Taipei Xian to study physics. In college he began the study of traditional Shaolin Long Fist (Changquan or Chang Chuan, 少林長拳) with Master Li, Mao-Ching at the Tamkang College Guoshu Club (淡江國術社) (1964–1968), and eventually became an assistant instructor under Master Li. In 1971 he completed his MS degree in physics at the National Taiwan University (台灣大學), and then served in the Chinese Air Force from 1971 to 1972. In the service, Dr. Yang taught physics at the Junior Academy of the Chinese Air Force (空軍幼校) while also teaching wushu. After being honorably discharged in 1972, he returned to Tamkang College to teach physics and resumed study under Master Li, Mao-Ching. From Master Li, Dr. Yang learned northern-style wushu, which includes both bare-hand (especially kicking) techniques and numerous weapons.

In 1974 Dr. Yang came to the United States to study mechanical engineering at Purdue University. At the request of a few students, Dr. Yang began to teach gongfu, which resulted in the foundation of the Purdue University Chinese Kung Fu Research Club in spring 1975. While at Purdue Dr. Yang also taught college-credited courses in taijiquan. In May 1978 he was awarded a PhD in mechanical engineering by Purdue.

In 1980 Dr. Yang moved to Houston to work for Texas Instruments. While in Houston he founded Yang's Shaolin Kung Fu Academy, which was eventually taken over by his disciple Mr. Jeffery Bolt after he moved to Boston in 1982. Dr. Yang founded Yang's Martial Arts Academy (YMAA) in Boston on October 1, 1982.

In January 1984 he gave up his engineering career to devote more time to research, writing, and teaching. In March 1986 he purchased property in the Jamaica Plain area of Boston to be used as the headquarters of the new organization, Yang's Martial Arts Association. The organization has continued to expand, and as of July 1, 1989, YMAA has become just one division of Yang's Oriental Arts Association, Inc. (YOAA, Inc.).

In summary, Dr. Yang has been involved in Chinese wushu since 1961. During this time, he has spent thirteen years learning Shaolin White Crane (Bai He), Shaolin Long Fist (Changquan), and taijiquan. Dr. Yang has more than twenty-seven years of instructional experience: seven years in Taiwan, five years at Purdue University, two years in Houston, Texas, and thirteen years in Boston, Massachusetts.

In addition, Dr. Yang has also been invited to offer seminars around the world to share his knowledge of Chinese martial arts and qigong. Countries he has visited include Canada, Mexico, France, Italy, Poland, England, Ireland, Portugal, Switzerland, Germany, Hungary, Spain, the Netherlands, Latvia, and Saudi Arabia.

Since 1986 YMAA has become an international organization that currently includes thirty-one schools located in Poland, Portugal, France, Latvia, Italy, the Netherlands, Hungary, South Africa, Saudi Arabia, Canada, Ireland, and the United States. Many of Dr. Yang's books and videos have been translated into French, Italian, Spanish, Polish, Czech, Bulgarian, and Hungarian.

Dr. Yang has published many other volumes on the martial arts and qigong:

1. *Shaolin Chin Na,* Unique Publications, Inc., 1980

2. *Shaolin Long Fist Kung Fu,* Unique Publications, Inc., 1981

3. *Yang Style Tai Chi Chuan,* Unique Publications, Inc., 1981

4. *Introduction to Ancient Chinese Weapons,* Unique Publications, Inc., 1985

5. *Ancient Chinese Weapons: A Martial Artist's Guide,* revised edition, YMAA Publication Center, 1999

6. *Chi Kung for Health and Martial Arts,* YMAA Publication Center, 1985

7. *Qigong—Health and Martial Arts,* revised edition, YMAA Publication Center, 1998

8. *Northern Shaolin Sword,* YMAA Publication Center, 1985

9. *Advanced Yang Style Tai Chi Chuan Vol. 1—Tai Chi Theory and Martial Power,* YMAA Publication Center, 1986

10. *Tai Chi Theory and Martial Power,* revised edition, YMAA Publication Center, 1996

11. *Advanced Yang Style Tai Chi Chuan Vol. 2—Tai Chi Chuan Martial Applications,* YMAA Publication Center, 1986

12. *Tai Chi Chuan Martial Applications,* revised edition, YMAA Publication Center, 1996

13. *Analysis of Shaolin Chin Na,* YMAA Publication Center, 1987, 2004

14. *The Eight Pieces of Brocade—Ba Duan Jin,* YMAA Publication Center, 1988

15. *Eight Simple Qigong Exercises for Health,* revised edition, YMAA Publication Center, 1997

16. *The Root of Chinese Qigong—The Secrets of Qigong Training,* YMAA Publication Center, 1989, 1997

17. *Muscle/Tendon Changing and Marrow/Brain Washing Chi Kung—The Secret of Youth,* YMAA Publication Center, 1989

18. *Qigong the Secret of Youth, Da Mo's Muscle Tendon Changing and Marrow Brain Washing Qigong,* revised edition, YMAA Publication Center, 2000

19. *Hsing Yi Chuan—Theory and Applications,* YMAA Publication Center, 1990

20. *Xingyiquan—Theory and Applications,* revised edition, YMAA Publication Center, 2003

21. *The Essence of Tai Chi Chi Kung—Health and Martial Arts,* YMAA Publication Center, 1990

22. *The Essence of Taiji Qigong—Health and Martial Arts,* revised edition, YMAA Publication Center, 1998

23. *Qigong for Arthritis,* YMAA Publication Center, 1991

24. *Arthritis Relief,* revised edition, YMAA Publication Center, 2005

25. *Chinese Qigong Massage—General Massage,* YMAA Publication Center, 1992

26. *Qigong Massage—Fundamental Techniques for Health and Relaxation,* revised edition, YMAA Publication Center, 2005

27. *How to Defend Yourself,* YMAA Publication Center, 1992

28. *Baguazhang—Emei Baguazhang,* YMAA Publication Center, 1994

29. *Baguazhang—Theory and Applications,* revised edition, YMAA Publication Center, 2008

30. *Comprehensive Applications of Shaolin Chin Na—The Practical Defense of Chinese Seizing Arts,* YMAA Publication Center, 1995

31. *Taiji Chin Na—The Seizing Art of Taijiquan,* YMAA Publication Center, 1995

32. *The Essence of Shaolin White Crane,* YMAA Publication Center, 1996

33. *Back Pain—Chinese Qigong for Healing and Prevention,* YMAA Publication Center, 1997

34. *Back Pain Relief—Chinese Qigong for Healing and Prevention,* revised edition, YMAA Publication Center, 2004

35. *Taijiquan Classical Yang Style—The Complete Form and Qigong,* YMAA Publication Center, 1999

36. *Tai Chi Chuan—Classical Yang Style,* revised edition, YMAA Publication Center, 2010

37. *Taijiquan Theory of Dr. Yang, Jwing-Ming—The Root of Taijiquan,* YMAA Publication Center, 2003

38. *Qigong Meditation—Embryonic Breathing,* YMAA Publication Center, 2003

39. *Qigong Meditation—Small Circulation,* YMAA Publication Center, 2006

40. *Tai Chi Ball Qigong—Health and Martial Arts,* YMAA Publication Center, 2010

Dr. Yang has also published the following DVDs:

1. *Chin Na in Depth Courses 1–4,* YMAA Publication Center, 2003

2. *Chin Na in Depth Courses 5–8,* YMAA Publication Center, 2003

3. *Chin Na in Depth Courses 9–12,* YMAA Publication Center, 2003

4. *Eight Simple Qigong Exercises for Health—The Eight Pieces of Brocade,* YMAA Publication Center, 2003

5. *Shaolin White Crane Gong Fu Basic Training Courses 1 & 2,* YMAA Publication Center, 2003

6. *Shaolin White Crane Hard and Soft Qigong,* YMAA Publication Center, 2003

7. *Taijiquan, Classical Yang Style (Long-Form Taijiquan),* YMAA Publication Center, 2003

8. *Analysis of Shaolin Chin Na,* YMAA Publication Center, 2004

9.   *Shaolin Kung Fu Fundamental Training*, YMAA Publication Center, 2004

10. *Baguazhang (Eight Trigrams Palm Kung Fu)*, YMAA Publication Center, 2005

11. *Essence of Taiji Qigong*, YMAA Publication Center, 2005

12. *Qigong Massage*, YMAA Publication Center, 2005

13. *Shaolin Long Fist Kung Fu Basic Sequences*, YMAA Publication Center, 2005

14. *Taiji Pushing Hands Courses 1 & 2*, YMAA Publication Center, 2005

15. *Taiji Sword, Classical Yang Style*, YMAA Publication Center, 2005

16. *Taiji Ball Qigong Courses 1 & 2*, YMAA Publication Center, 2006

17. *Taiji Fighting Set—88 Posture, 2-Person Matching Set*, YMAA Publication Center, 2006

18. *Taiji Pushing Hands Courses 3 & 4*, YMAA Publication Center, 2006

19. *Understanding Qigong DVD 1—What Is Qigong? Understanding the Human Qi Circulatory System*, YMAA Publication Center, 2006

20. *Understanding Qigong DVD 2—Keypoints of Qigong & Qigong Breathing*, YMAA Publication Center, 2006

21. *Shaolin Saber Basic Sequences*, YMAA Publication Center, 2007

22. *Shaolin Staff Basic Sequences*, YMAA Publication Center, 2007

23. *Simple Qigong Exercises for Arthritis Relief*, YMAA Publication Center, 2007

24. *Simple Qigong Exercises for Back Pain Relief*, YMAA Publication Center, 2007

25. *Taiji & Shaolin Staff Fundamental Training*, YMAA Publication Center, 2007

26. *Taiji Ball Qigong Courses 3 & 4*, YMAA Publication Center, 2007

27. *Understanding Qigong DVD 3—Embryonic Breathing*, YMAA Publication Center, 2007

28. *Understanding Qigong DVD 4—Four Seasons Qigong*, YMAA Publication Center, 2007

29. *Understanding Qigong DVD 5—Small Circulation*, YMAA Publication Center, 2007

30. *Understanding Qigong DVD 6—Martial Arts Qigong Breathing*, YMAA Publication Center, 2007

31. *Five Animal Sports Qigong*, YMAA Publication Center, 2008

32. *Saber Fundamental Training*, YMAA Publication Center, 2008

33. *Shaolin White Crane Gong Fu Basic Training Courses 3 & 4*, YMAA Publication Center, 2008

34. *Taiji 37 Postures Martial Applications*, YMAA Publication Center, 2008

35. *Taiji Saber, Classical Yang Style*, YMAA Publication Center, 2008

36. *Taiji Wrestling—Advanced Takedown Techniques,* YMAA Publication Center, 2008

37. *Taiji Yin/Yang Sticking Hands,* YMAA Publication Center, 2008

38. *Xingyiquan (Hsing I Chuan),* YMAA Publication Center, 2008

39. *Northern Shaolin Sword,* YMAA Publication Center, 2009

40. *Sword Fundamental Training,* YMAA Publication Center, 2009

41. *Taiji Chin Na in Depth,* YMAA Publication Center, 2009

42. *YMAA 25-Year Anniversary,* YMAA Publication Center, 2009

43. *Shuai Jiao—Kung Fu Wrestling,* YMAA Publication Center, 2010

BOOKS FROM YMAA

101 REFLECTIONS ON TAI CHI CHUAN
108 INSIGHTS INTO TAI CHI CHUAN
A SUDDEN DAWN: THE EPIC JOURNEY OF BODHIDHARMA
A WOMAN'S QIGONG GUIDE
ADVANCING IN TAE KWON DO
ANALYSIS OF SHAOLIN CHIN NA 2ND ED
ANCIENT CHINESE WEAPONS
THE ART AND SCIENCE OF STAFF FIGHTING
ART OF HOJO UNDO
ARTHRITIS RELIEF, 3D ED.
BACK PAIN RELIEF, 2ND ED.
BAGUAZHANG, 2ND ED.
BRAIN FITNESS
CARDIO KICKBOXING ELITE
CHIN NA IN GROUND FIGHTING
CHINESE FAST WRESTLING
CHINESE FITNESS
CHINESE TUI NA MASSAGE
CHOJUN
COMPLETE MARTIAL ARTIST
COMPREHENSIVE APPLICATIONS OF SHAOLIN CHIN NA
CONFLICT COMMUNICATION
CROCODILE AND THE CRANE: A NOVEL
CUTTING SEASON: A XENON PEARL MARTIAL ARTS THRILLER
DAO DE JING
DAO IN ACTION
DEFENSIVE TACTICS
DESHI: A CONNOR BURKE MARTIAL ARTS THRILLER
DIRTY GROUND
DR. WU'S HEAD MASSAGE
DUKKHA HUNGRY GHOSTS
DUKKHA REVERB
DUKKHA, THE SUFFERING: AN EYE FOR AN EYE
DUKKHA UNLOADED
ENZAN: THE FAR MOUNTAIN, A CONNOR BURKE MARTIAL ARTS
    THRILLER
ESSENCE OF SHAOLIN WHITE CRANE
EVEN IF IT KILLS ME
EXPLORING TAI CHI
FACING VIOLENCE
FIGHT BACK
FIGHT LIKE A PHYSICIST
THE FIGHTER'S BODY
FIGHTER'S FACT BOOK
FIGHTER'S FACT BOOK 2
THE FIGHTING ARTS
FIGHTING THE PAIN RESISTANT ATTACKER
FIRST DEFENSE
FORCE DECISIONS: A CITIZENS GUIDE
FOX BORROWS THE TIGER'S AWE
INSIDE TAI CHI
THE JUDO ADVANTAGE
THE JUJI GATAME ENCYCLOPEDIA
KAGE: THE SHADOW, A CONNOR BURKE MARTIAL ARTS THRILLER
KARATE SCIENCE
KATA AND THE TRANSMISSION OF KNOWLEDGE
KRAV MAGA COMBATIVES
KRAV MAGA PROFESSIONAL TACTICS
KRAV MAGA WEAPON DEFENSES
LITTLE BLACK BOOK OF VIOLENCE
LIUHEBAFA FIVE CHARACTER SECRETS
MARTIAL ARTS ATHLETE
MARTIAL ARTS INSTRUCTION
MARTIAL WAY AND ITS VIRTUES
MASK OF THE KING
MEDITATIONS ON VIOLENCE
MERIDIAN QIGONG EXERCISES
MIND/BODY FITNESS
MINDFUL EXERCISE
THE MIND INSIDE TAI CHI
THE MIND INSIDE YANG STYLE TAI CHI CHUAN
MUGAI RYU
NATURAL HEALING WITH QIGONG
NORTHERN SHAOLIN SWORD, 2ND ED.
OKINAWA'S COMPLETE KARATE SYSTEM: ISSHIN RYU
THE PAIN-FREE BACK

PAIN-FREE JOINTS
POWER BODY
PRINCIPLES OF TRADITIONAL CHINESE MEDICINE
THE PROTECTOR ETHIC
QIGONG FOR HEALTH & MARTIAL ARTS 2ND ED.
QIGONG FOR LIVING
QIGONG FOR TREATING COMMON AILMENTS
QIGONG MASSAGE
QIGONG MEDITATION: EMBRYONIC BREATHING
QIGONG MEDITATION: SMALL CIRCULATION
QIGONG, THE SECRET OF YOUTH: DA MO'S CLASSICS
QUIET TEACHER: A XENON PEARL MARTIAL ARTS THRILLER
RAVEN'S WARRIOR
REDEMPTION
ROOT OF CHINESE QIGONG, 2ND ED.
SAMBO ENCYCLOPEDIA
SCALING FORCE
SELF-DEFENSE FOR WOMEN
SENSEI: A CONNOR BURKE MARTIAL ARTS THRILLER
SHIHAN TE: THE BUNKAI OF KATA
SHIN GI TAI: KARATE TRAINING FOR BODY, MIND, AND SPIRIT
SIMPLE CHINESE MEDICINE
SIMPLE QIGONG EXERCISES FOR HEALTH, 3RD ED.
SIMPLIFIED TAI CHI CHUAN, 2ND ED.
SOLO TRAINING
SOLO TRAINING 2
SUMO FOR MIXED MARTIAL ARTS
SUNRISE TAI CHI
SUNSET TAI CHI
SURVIVING ARMED ASSAULTS
TAE KWON DO: THE KOREAN MARTIAL ART
TAEKWONDO BLACK BELT POOMSAE
TAEKWONDO: A PATH TO EXCELLENCE
TAEKWONDO: ANCIENT WISDOM FOR THE MODERN WARRIOR
TAEKWONDO: DEFENSE AGAINST WEAPONS
TAEKWONDO: SPIRIT AND PRACTICE
TAO OF BIOENERGETICS
TAI CHI BALL QIGONG: FOR HEALTH AND MARTIAL ARTS
TAI CHI BALL WORKOUT FOR BEGINNERS
THE TAI CHI BOOK
TAI CHI CHIN NA: THE SEIZING ART OF TAI CHI CHUAN,
    2ND ED.
TAI CHI CHUAN CLASSICAL YANG STYLE, 2ND ED.
TAI CHI CHUAN MARTIAL POWER, 3RD ED.
TAI CHI CONNECTIONS
TAI CHI DYNAMICS
TAI CHI FOR DEPRESSION
TAI CHI IN 10 WEEKS
TAI CHI QIGONG, 3RD ED.
TAI CHI SECRETS OF THE ANCIENT MASTERS
TAI CHI SECRETS OF THE WU & LI STYLES
TAI CHI SECRETS OF THE WU STYLE
TAI CHI SECRETS OF THE YANG STYLE
TAI CHI SWORD: CLASSICAL YANG STYLE, 2ND ED.
TAI CHI SWORD FOR BEGINNERS
TAI CHI WALKING
TAIJIQUAN THEORY OF DR. YANG, JWING-MING
TAO OF BIOENERGETICS
TENGU: THE MOUNTAIN GOBLIN, A CONNOR BURKE MARTIAL ARTS
    THRILLER
TIMING IN THE FIGHTING ARTS
TRADITIONAL CHINESE HEALTH SECRETS
TRADITIONAL TAEKWONDO
TRAINING FOR SUDDEN VIOLENCE
TRUE WELLNESS
TRUE WELLNESS: THE MIND
THE WARRIOR'S MANIFESTO
WAY OF KATA
WAY OF KENDO AND KENJITSU
WAY OF SANCHIN KATA
WAY TO BLACK BELT
WESTERN HERBS FOR MARTIAL ARTISTS
WILD GOOSE QIGONG
WINNING FIGHTS
WISDOM'S WAY
XINGYIQUAN

DVDS FROM YMAA

more products available from . . .
YMAA Publication Center, Inc. 楊氏東方文化出版中心
1-800-669-8892 • info@ymaa.com • www.ymaa.com

Lightning Source UK Ltd.
Milton Keynes UK
UKHW031357160922
408974UK00018B/312